Super-Vision

*Recommendations of the Consensus Conference
of Midwifery Supervision*

Association of Radical Midwives

Books for Midwives Press
in conjunction with the
Association of Radical Midwives

Published by Books for Midwives Press, 174a Ashley Road, Hale, Cheshire, WA15 9SF, England

© 1995, Association of Radical Midwives

First edition

ISBN 1-898507-34-1

British Library Cataloguing in Publication Data
A catalogue record for this book is available from the British Library

Printed in Great Britain by Cromwell Press Ltd

Contents

Preface

More than a Conference Report, this book contains a c
the speakers at the Conference in which they exp
recommendations for future midwifery supervision and
Mayes who chaired the afternoon session.

The speakers were drawn from a wide range of midwifery fields – clinical practice, management, supervision, research, education, as well as other disciplines such as social work and psychotherapy.

During the Conference the delegates formed six discussion groups, each exploring a different aspect of the topic and putting forward their recommendations for improvements in Midwifery supervision.

The idea for the Conference sprang from the work of the ARM Working Party which was set up in response to the apparent increase in midwives being disciplined, either informally or officially. In too many cases the quality of midwifery supervision gave cause for concern. Various reasons were put forward, including the difficulties inherent in the dual role of manager/supervisor required of most of the midwifery managers in the UK.

Introduction

For and against midwifery supervision

A debate during the ARM National Meeting in March 1993 which led to the conference

It was unanimously agreed that this is a topic requiring extensive debate, but in the short time left before the main speaker, we decided to hear two differing views, put forward by Caroline Flint and Soo Downe.

Caroline Flint believes that supervision of midwifery can be an oppressive tool. She told us that she is often contacted by midwives who have been accused of having done something wrong, and although the case may not go as far as actual disciplinary action, colleagues are aware that this particular midwife has been 'called to the office' as it were, and in many cases the midwife never gets a chance to clear her name. Quite frequently it is an issue of clinical judgement on which supervisor and midwife disagree. Caroline feels strongly that as a profession, we should not allow our clinical judgement to be challenged in this way, retrospectively and with no opportunity for open debate on the matter. We have an unfortunate tendency to make retrospective criticism of other people's clinical judgement. The important issue is what we do at the time, given the circumstances and with all the resources we have available at that moment. Sometimes we will make mistakes. There is no question about this, but as a profession we should be able to make a clinical judgement, which perhaps others would not have made, but was actually alright. A clinical decision may be questioned, but should not be criticized, and even less should be the cause for supervisory action.

Caroline believes midwifery suffers from the 'nursing' model, which says there is only one 'right' way of doing things, which actually doesn't work when dealing with people in a clinical situation. She agreed that good supervision can be a lifeline, especially in the present climate of change in the NHS, but she firmly believes it is a millstone round our neck. Even the word 'supervisor' has caused problems, it is so open to misinterpretation, by non-midwives and even those within midwifery. As an independent midwife working in many different Health Authorities, Caroline said she has over 100 supervisors who feel they can supervise her practice, and she feels this is wrong.

Soo Downe is concerned that there is no machinery for appealing against an accusation made by a supervisor which does not subsequently get a hearing at a higher level. She believes that supervision is a powerful tool, but that it should be restrained by a system of appeal.

She agreed that a lot of what Caroline had said was very valid. However, she reminded us that doctors have got away with a lot of bad practice on the basis of clinical judgement. She said there should be some method of clinical audit, however it is set up. We have to get away from saying, 'we're the experts, you can't challenge us'. Our practice must be open to challenge.

Standards of supervision vary, and Soo said that she was coming from a different situation from Caroline's, as supervision is working very well in her Health Authority, and as far as she is aware midwives are only referred to the ENB for valid reasons. The word 'practitioner' catches all those who practice and the supervisor has a role in ensuring an accepted standard of practice for everyone.

The difficulty lies in the way complaints are handled. For instance, the supervisor refers the case to the link supervisor, who refers it to Regional level. If at this stage the decision is that it should go no further, that's that – end of story. This is most unsatisfactory, as the midwife in question has not really had her name cleared.

We need a system whereby if a midwife feels she has been wrongly accused, she should be able to go to a peer group, or an Expert Committee of midwives, who will then look at the evidence, look at the outcome, check the research, examine the conditions under which the midwife was employed, the situation at the time, the education etc. and decide whether in this case the accusation was appropriate or not.

Following these two speakers, a general discussion followed, with several pertinent points being brought out including; the power of a Supervisor to modify or veto, on grounds of practice standards, changes being brought about in the present upheaval of the NHS and the new requirement for adequate training as a Supervisor where previously the post was almost an automatic adjunct to a managerial position following a scanty few days instruction. A few members cited the innovative appointment of E and F grade midwives as Supervisors.

The general feeling was that perhaps ARM should form a working party to examine the whole concept, then issue a consensus statement, saying 'this is what we want'. Initially the debate will be opened up within *Midwifery Matters* and other journals, and individuals wishing to form a Working Party can then come forward at the next National Meeting.

The Supervision Working Party was formed and began work in the Autumn of 1993, producing 'Draft Proposals for Midwifery Supervision' in the Spring of 1994, in response to which the Consensus Conference was held in April 1995.

The History of Midwifery Supervision

Mavis Kirkham

In order to understand the factors affecting the supervision of midwives now, it is useful to look at where we came from in terms of both the legislation and the social factors that have influenced supervision in practice.

There have always been social tensions around the control of midwifery. The midwife who inspires self confidence in childbearing women has a powerful skill. Where women have a lowly position in society that power is likely to be seen as subversive. Many women have suffered for this and the powerholders in society have sought to control them.

In Tudor times the first formal arrangements for the control of midwives in England required them to swear before the Bishop's court to 'faithfully and diligently exercise the office' of midwife and use no 'sorcery or incantations'. The church did not have direct entry to the women's world of the lying in chamber and so midwives were required to produce 'six honest matrons' whom they had delivered during their period of instruction who would testify to their skill (Donnison, 1977). Thus the first Act to register midwives emphasized their mutual dependence with the women of their community.

Things had changed a lot by the nineteenth century in terms of occupational specialization and social power. Services around childbearing and health had moved from the domestic world of women to the male market arena (Witz, 1992). Whilst most care around childbirth continued to be provided by local women known to all those they cared for, a very different group sought to make midwifery a profession fit for ladies.

The Matron's Aid Society changed its name in 1886 to the Midwives Institute, it later becoming the Royal College of Midwives. To the early members of the Midwives Institute the raising of the social standing of midwifery was very closely linked with the aim of improving standards of midwifery care by the registration of midwives.

Historical studies show that status within occupational structures does not rest on technical skills alone but is supported by members' social origins in 'groups already enjoying high status and power in society' (Elliot, 1972). Such status was never held by the average midwife who was poor, often illiterate and working irregularly. The Midwives Institute, however, represented 'not the whole of midwifery but the views and interests of the elite leadership' (Haegerty, 1990), a group of Victorian ladies.

The early members of the Midwives Institute trained in the most prestigious midwifery courses but few continued in clinical practice after qualification. They immediately moved into the highest positions of management in maternity and philanthropic institutions as befitted their position in society. The social gap between the ladies of the Institute and the practising midwives was immense.

To add to this the midwife members of the Institute's council were all trained nurses and nursing training, in this era, strictly instilled deference to male medical authority.

> 'Every medical man has a right to look for loyalty, a steady upholding of his authority to the patient... and the remembrance of the nurse that she is there to do what she is told, and not either to give, or to try to carry out her own opinions.' (Nursing Notes, November, 1900: 156)

The leadership believed midwifery to be 'the inferior branch of the healing profession' and medicine to be midwifery's 'natural leader and superior' (Nursing Notes, April 1915: 182).

The struggle for higher training and status for midwifery and therefore for state registration was set within the hierarchical structure of Victorian society. Women did not have the resources to achieve change. They therefore worked by proxy through sympathetic men. They did this with a skill highly developed in reforming Victorian ladies and not unknown in midwives today.

The supporters of the 1902 Act sought to preserve the role of the midwife as an independent practitioner within the strictly defined sphere of normal childbearing. Such a role would relieve doctors of 'tiresome and unrenumerative work' (HMSO, 1892: 22). This fitted the world view of many of the aristocrats of British medicine who saw midwifery as 'an occupation degrading to a gentleman' (Smith, 1979: 23).

In this situation the boundaries between midwifery and medicine had to be clearly set. 'What you want to educate midwives for is for them to know their own ignorance. This is really the one great object in educating midwives' (HMSO, 1892: 101). Midwifery education was to be 'kept necessarily and designedly limited' (HMSO 1892: 121). The boundaries of midwifery were thus drawn by medicine in what has been described as 'a demarcationary strategy of deskilling' (Witz, 1992:112).

1902 Midwives Act

This Act is usually seen as the foundation stone of modern midwifery. Without it we would not be here today. It was also the product of the Victorian society which produced it and this has left a deep mark upon midwifery and its supervision.

The Act set up the statutory body, the Central Midwives Board. Midwifery thus achieved,

'...the unenviable distinction of being the only profession controlled by a body on which its members must never be more than a minority.' (Donnison, 1977, p.179.)

Until 1920 membership of the CMB was not actually required to include midwives at all, although women were allowed to be members from the beginning.

The inspection of midwives

After the 1902 Act the leaders of midwifery continued to seek to raise the status of the profession. Meanwhile most practising midwives were very much part of the working class community which they served. Routine inspection of midwives was carried out across this large social divide. There was no training for inspectors nor were they required to be midwives and many Local Supervising Authorities preferred 'a lady' who would be used to supervising subordinates. This led to much misunderstanding particularly with young ladies inspecting very experienced midwives.

'...the midwife herself was expected to conform to the moral and cultural standards of middle class social reformers, rather than those of the working class community in which most midwives had their roots. From this framework of stipulations and restrictions would emerge the ideal midwife: one who was no longer placed the women she attended before her submission to the medical profession and her deference to her social betters.' (Haegerty 1990:82)

Nursing Notes (June, 1907: 89) recommended that midwives 'should avoid any rough work, such as scrubbing, grate cleaning or polishing' in their domestic lives. In reality few midwives could afford not to do this work themselves. Some midwives were deemed to be unclean by the lady inspector who visited their home unannounced when, far from practising as midwives, they were cleaning the grate. Similarly Nursing Notes (July 1907: 106, August 1907:121) warned midwives to 'use plenty of clean linen' and 'insist on cleanliness on the part of the patient'. The cases of the CMB Penal Committee (Heagarty, 1990) include many appeals by midwives to the CMB on the grounds that their patient just did not possess the required clean linen. Midwives were in a similarly impossible position when caring for families where the rules required that they summon medical aid and the family's poverty meant they could not pay the doctor's fee. In this era many midwives' 'offences' were caused by their poverty and their respect for the poverty of those in their care. Many midwives were struck off the Role for those reasons despite long petitions on their behalf.

Not only was the inspection of midwives experienced as punitive but the disciplinary procedure was weighed against the midwife:

'The Board endowed itself and the LSA's with almost unlimited authority over the women they supervised. The Rules stipulated that the LSA's were free to investigate any aspect of the midwife's practice, from following her on her rounds, to questioning her patients, to investigating her living arrangements and her personal life... the greater burden of proof fell on the midwife and not the authorities. The Rules freed the LSA's and the Board from having to act only on judicial rules of evidence. The Board strengthened its ability to convict accused midwives by allowing hearsay as a valid form of evidence. Probably most indicative of the Board's power lay in its relationship to the entire process itself. The Board not only formally charged the midwife and prosecuted her but it judged her as well.' (Haegarty, 1990: 83)

Even within this framework it cannot be said that inspection was wholly destructive. The Medical Officer of Health for Northamptonshire, for example, reported to the CMB,

'Though not used to technical terms, it astonished me very often the amount of practical knowledge they possess, and the self-reliance they show. Most of them always welcome being shown and told better methods than their own though, of course some of them are quite illiterate and think the midwives Act all fuss, they nevertheless endeavour to comply to the rules.' (CMB,1914)

Nor can it be said that the life of an Inspector was easy and Nursing Notes contains accounts of the problems of teaching illiterate midwives to use clinical thermometers. The problems of record keeping were also great 'as in many cases the writing has to be done by relatives'. (Lancashire LSA reported in Nursing Notes March, 1907 p.40)

Many bona fide midwives continued to practice and the key argument against them – that their practice put childbearing women at risk of infection – was not substantiated. One unusually perceptive Inspector of Midwives surveyed her 1907-1918 statistics and found 'the figures show the lowest death rates amongst mothers attended by the very women that the Midwives Act 1902 was passed to do away with' (Nursing Notes, March 1931).

Nevertheless the campaign against the bona fide midwife continued 'The handywoman was derided as the arch enemy of midwifery throughout the late 1920s and 1930s and articles in Nursing Notes demonstrate the fervour of the campaign.' (Leap, Hunter, 1993). It is said of the 1926 Act that,

'though not as strong as we wished, there is evidence that it can be an efficient weapon against the deprecations of our foe "the handylady"'. (Nursing Notes, January 1928)

I have long puzzled over why the Inspectors of Midwives were so punitive towards working class midwives at a time when the Lady Factory Inspectors were so enlightened (McFeely, 1988). Factory workers were a clearly separate social group whom their inspectors sought to protect. Midwives were much more socially problematic. They had to be controlled because their practice was perceived as a potential threat to medical practice on the one hand whilst on the other hand being 'with women' in working class practice was perceived as a threat to midwifery leaders' aspirations to raise the status of midwifery to that of a profession. Ironically that status could only be raised by subservience to the medical powerholders. Thus the non-medical inspectors, in many different senses policed midwifery on behalf of the medical profession.

As time passed some of the factors separating Inspectors and midwives changed and the gap between them narrowed. The payment by the local authority to GPs (1918) when called by a midwife greatly helped poor families and improved the midwife's chance of getting paid for that case. Monetary compensation (1926) for midwives suspended from practice after contact with infection was a great help to poor midwives and their families.

The 1936 Midwives Act required LSAs to provide a salaried midwifery service. From this point supervision and management, whilst separate functions in law, were often difficult to separate in practice. This problem grew as managerial hierarchies developed.

The 1937 Ministry of Health Letter is significant in that it acknowledged many of the problems being experienced with supervision and sought to remedy them. The Letter acknowledged the 'bad psychological effect upon the midwife' of being supervised by a non-midwife. Supervisors were therefore required to have 'adequate experience in the practice of midwifery'. Some social distance was presumably thought to be required when it was stressed that 'it is not desirable for a Supervisor of Midwives to be engaged in the actual practice of midwifery'. The Letter stated that an Inspector of Midwives should be regarded as 'the counsellor and friend of the midwife, rather than a relentless critic'. She should also have 'sympathy and tact' and be called a Supervisor rather than an Inspector.

Paragraph seven extended supervisors to cover all midwives including those working in hospital and distinction was made between the supervision and management of salaried midwives.

Nevertheless, whilst the Letter stated problems and sought to solve them the problems were political as well as 'psychological' and the issues of power and control were not addressed. It was important to raise midwife's need for a 'counsellor and friend' but the supervisor also had a policing role. These are two potentially opposing roles and containing them both within the function of supervision inevitably led to problems.

Various acts and regulations have sought to ensure that supervisors have both the experience and the education to fit them for the role of 'counsellor and friend'. Yet the dilemma remains that at the same time she is required to review standards of practice and advise the LSA in situations where there may be professional misconduct.

The Midwives Act 1951 continued to link supervision with the control of midwives. The Board was stated to have the power to make rules 'regulating, supervising and restricting within due limits the practice of midwives'. Supervisors were also required to ensure that midwives attended statutory refresher courses.

The 1974 National Health Service (Re-organization) Act

This first organization of the NHS brought hospital, community and other services together into unified Health Authorities. District midwives became employees of the health authorities rather than the local authorities. Regional Health Authorities were nominated as LSAs and supervisors were nominated by the District Health Authorities and approved by the LSAs. As supervision moved away from the Medical Officer of

Health and senior district midwives it ceased to be within a public health framework which was concerned with many other aspects of women's lives and health such as public housing. In 1977 the requirement for a medical supervisor of midwives was abolished. Midwives were therefore supervised by midwives but largely supervised within hospitals and the hierarchical framework of health authorities. It can be argued (Alison, 1995) that from this time supervision had an institutional and professional context only, it lacked a context in public health or the lives of childbearing women.

The 1974 and 1977 changes in the context and organization of supervision were very important. Parallel processes can be seen in midwifery: as we are cared for so do we care for women, as we are managed so do we manage our clients. If this is so, then the move of supervision into such hierarchical structures was very significant. It is deeply ironic that supervision gained a hierarchy and lost a social context just when it came under midwifery control for the first time.

The 1979 Nurses, Midwives and Health Visitors Act abolished the CMB and created the United Kingdom Central Council for Nursing, Midwifery and Health Visiting and the National Boards which served the three professions. Ironically, the CMB had a majority of midwife members just before its abolition (Bent, 1995). The new statutory bodies can never have a majority of midwife members as they serve three professions. Both the UKCC and the Boards were required to have a midwifery committee whose advice concerning midwifery was to be listened to but not necessarily acted upon.

The wording of the 1979 Act continued to identify supervision with the control of midwives.

What is supervision for?

In its early years supervision was clearly concerned with the control of midwives. 'Supervision was the mechanism introduced to ensure compliance with the statutory regulations amongst a self-employed group who were often isolated' (Jenkins, 1995). This compliance was clearly felt to be crucial by those who held power over or within midwifery at that time. Now midwives are controlled in very different ways,

> 'Midwives are for the most part employees; communications systems are rapid and very powerful; most midwives work in large and controlled establishments (hospitals) and those who work in the community are usually managed from the hospital base. Yet there has been almost no change in the statutory requirements.' (Jenkins, 1995)

The Midwives Rules require all LSAs to publish 'details of how midwives will be supervised'. These documents vary. Rosmary Jenkins (1995) has identified a 'core of work' which is common to all. (This list of tasks is reproduced at the end of the list of Key Events in the Supervision of Midwives in England p.14). The nature of these tasks demonstrates the different and sometimes potentially contradictory aspects of the supervisors role.

Some of these tasks are administrative and scarcely merit the title of supervisory. This is the case with the collection and collation of midwives intention to practice notices, though supervisors need to know who they are to supervise.

Some of these tasks are concerned with audit and inspection such as the regular supervisory visits to each midwife to review her standards of practice and record keeping, to audit her drug records and inspect her premises where necessary. The extent to which this audit is conducted in a supportive manner is determined by the supervisor herself.

Some of the supervisor's tasks are concerned with the policing of the profession namely in advising the LSA in situations where suspension from practice and referral to the UKCC are being considered by the LSA. Whilst these latter acts can only be done by the LSA they are widely perceived as the LSA end of a continuum of supervision. The rest of the continuum is seen to consist of supervisory interviews within which the individual supervisor has considerable power. She may choose to share that power with the midwife but the midwife has no right of appeal against supervisory decisions.

Some of the tasks of the supervisor are concerned with professional support being available to midwives to discuss practice issues. The 1994 Code of Practice stresses this issue around, for instance, home births where there is no medical support. In this area too the supervisor has considerable power. An increasing number of supervisors seek to be a true friend and counsellor to midwives reclaiming their autonomy. Yet the dilemmas of the role are exemplified by press reports where supervisors appear to be supporting the midwife in opposing her client's choice (e.g. Smith, 1994) or blocking the midwife who seeks to support her client's choice. The 1994 Code of Practice stresses the 'positive working relationship' (paragraph 51) between midwife and supervisor to 'work towards the common aim of optimum care for mothers and babies' (paragraph 49). The supervisor is concerned with 'safety in practice and care' and the supervisor is assumed to have the power to define what is safe. The supervisor certainly assumed that power in the case cited above (Smith, 1994).

Other supervisory tasks are educational in terms of assessing training needs, identifying new skills needed and facilitating appropriate training as well as ensuring that midwives attend refresher courses. In the modern era of life long learning this aspect of the supervisor's role can be seen as providing professional support and facilitating the midwife in assessing her own educational needs.

Management and supervision

The 1937 statement that a supervisor should be experienced in midwifery but not currently practising has not been observed for many years. Supervisors need to be aware of current issues in midwifery and in times of rapid change this means current practice. In a hierarchical health service the authority of the supervisor's role has been identified with the authority of management.

It is ironic that early supervision may have been autocratic in its operation but it is not hierarchical in its own structures. After 1974 supervision moved into large and hierarchical structures. The creation of link supervisors who were 'not taking a recognized superior role but nevertheless acting in a leadership capacity' (Jenkins, 1995) built a further hierarchical level into supervision. There is something ironic about one's 'counsellor and friend' being not just imposed but hierarchically organized.

Most supervisors now hold management positions. A manager's role is to organize a workforce on behalf of an employer. The identification of management with supervision has brought further complexity to the role of the supervisor. If the role of public watchdog and professional supporter are difficult to combine, the additional role of employer's advocate adds further potential role conflict. There have been many examples of supervisors not understanding the difference between the roles of supervisor and manager and of policy documents being based on this confusion (Beech, 1993).

It is difficult for a midwife in difficulties to seek out a 'counsellor and friend' if that person is identified with her employer as her manager. This is made more difficult with modern management practices. Can a midwife on a short term contract discuss her practice with self-awareness as to her shortcomings with the manager she will shortly meet for Individual Performance Review? There are also problems in terms of confidentiality (Beech, 1993).

Supervisors do not have to be managers and the 1994 revision of the Midwives Code of Practice (paragraph 47) states that a supervisor should be an 'experienced midwife' not a 'senior experienced midwife' as previously stated. There are now some F grade supervisors but overall supervision is still closely identified with management. With the hierarchical nature of the NHS, is this inevitable? Is it desirable?

We have had midwifery supervision for a long time and there have been great changes. The supervision of midwives has improved. The potential conflicts within the role of supervisor still remain. The shadow of the Inspector and the reality of the manager are still experienced by the midwife in supervision.

As I understand it, the difference between 'clinical supervision' which other professionals have and 'general supervision' in midwifery lies in the sense in which the supervisor of midwives acts in the wider interests of childbearing women. The question of whether a public watchdog can also be a professional friend (Isherwood, 1988) has not been sufficiently addressed. Our watchdogs are now required to be well trained (UKCC, 1994), some are friendly, supportive and innovative. Some of the terminology around the role has changed and midwives now have much more in common with their supervisors than was the case earlier this century. The UKCC has endeavoured to foster this common ground.

If there is a need for a watchdog on behalf of childbearing women, we must audit whether supervision effectively provides such a service. In the past, supervisors have been accused of witch hunting rather than effective audit. As we strive to build a more sensitive service, we may also need a 'counsellor and friend' who provides therapeutic supervision to help us develop real awareness of our own needs and those of others and plan to meet those needs. Our service must make available the skilled help and the time for such development. When midwifery was a new profession these roles were combined. One question that led to the calling of this conference is this – at the end of the twentieth century, are midwives sufficiently mature as a profession to chose our own friends?

References

Allison, J. (1995). Personal Communication.

Association of Supervisors of Midwives (1992). *Supervision – The Whys and Wherefores*. Great Yarmouth: ASM.

Beech, B.L. (1993). 'Supervision of midwives'. *Aims Journal* 5:2 pp.1–3.

Bent, A. (1995). Personal Communication.

Donnison, J. (1977). *Midwives and Medical Men*. London: Heinemann.

Heagerty, B.V (1990). *Gender and Professionalization: The Struggle for British Midwifery 1900–1936*. unpublished Phd thesis, Michigan State University. (copy in RCM library, London)

HMSO (1892). *Report from the Select Committee on the Registration of Midwives, House of Commons*. London: HMSO.

Isherwood, K (1988). 'Friend or watchdog?' *Nursing Times* 84:24 June 15th. p.65.

Jenkins, R. (1995). *The Law and Midwifery*. Oxford: Blackwell

Leap, N., Hunter, B. (1993). *The Midwife's Tale*. London: Scarlet Press.

McFeeley, M.D. (1988). *Lady Inspectors*. Oxford: Blackwell.

Nursing Notes archives kept in RCM library London.

Royal College of Midwives (1991). *Report of the Royal College of Midwives Commission on Legislation Relating to Midwives*. London: RCM.

Smith, J. (1994). 'We told you so'. *Aims Journal* 6:3 pp.10–12.

Smith, F.B (1979). *The People's Health*. London: Croom Helm.

UKCC (1994). *A Midwife's Code of Practice*. London: UKCC.

Witz, A. (1992). *Professions and Patriarchy*. London: Routledge.

Key Events in the History of the Supervision of Midwives in England

1902 Midwives Act

The Act set up the statutory body, the Central Midwives Board which had a medical majority.

The CMB was required to:

1. Institute training
2. Register midwives, including bona fides midwives
3. Issue and withdraw certificates
4. Establish and maintain a Roll of Practising Midwives
5. Define and limit the midwife's sphere of practice
6. Discipline midwives who disobeyed or ignored the Rules or who were guilty of negligence, malpractice or misconduct, the latter being personal as well as professional

The CMB delegated supervising and monitoring to Local Supervising Authorities which until 1974 were County Councils and County Borough Councils.

The LSA was to:
1. Exercise general supervision of midwives practising within their area (few, if any, were employed)
2. Investigate charges of misconduct, negligence or malpractice and report to the CMB
3. Report a midwife convicted of an offence
4. Suspend from practice midwives who were likely to be a source of infection
5. Require midwives to notify their intention to practice and submit a Roll of Midwives to the CMB annually
6. Report the death of a midwife
7. Report to the CMB the effect of the Act

These requirements have altered only slightly since 1902 though some things have been added.

The LSAs performed their functions via a Midwifery Committee on which women were allowed to sit and which would almost certainly include the Medical Officer of Health. The Medical Officer was mainly responsible for 'general supervision' and appointed a non-medical supervisor to undertake the bulk of the work and to be responsible to him. The non-medical supervisor was usually a non-midwife, sometimes a Health Visitor but always a lady. The supervisors, medical and non-medical were called Inspectors of Midwives.

The Institute of Inspectors of Midwives was formed in 1910.

The 1910 Midwives Act allowed no further issuing of certificates to bona fide midwives. They could only be awarded after successful completion of an approved course of training. Bona fide midwives already practising could continue.

The 1918 Act required midwives to notify the LSA via the Supervisor of Midwives, when medical aid had been summoned. Thus the GP could be paid by the LSA.

The 1926 Act allowed the suspension of midwives from the practice if liable to be a source of, or in contact with, infection and enabled monetary compensation during suspension. The supervisor notified the LSA of such suspensions. The Act also banned men or uncertified women from attending women in childbirth except under the direct and formal supervision of a duly qualified medical practitioner unless there was a sudden emergency. The last bona fide midwife only left the Role in 1947 (Leap and Hunter, 1993).

The 1936 Act stated that a salaried service had to be provided by the LSA to meet the needs of the local population. Some LSAs had been doing this for some years but 'now it was mandatory and managing midwives became a function separate from supervision' (ASM, 1992).

The Ministry of Health Letter 1937
This letter is of such importance that it is quoted in full.

Sir,

(1) I am directed by the Minister of Health to enclose for the information of the Council copies of the Regulations which he has made under Section 9 (2) of the Midwives Act, 1936, prescribing the qualifications of persons appointed by Local Supervising Authorities under Section 8 of the Midwives Act, 1902, to exercise supervision over midwives practising in their areas. The Regulations, which have been made after consultation with the Central Midwives Board and the Association of Local Authorities concerned, will come into operation on the 1st June next.

(2) It will be observed that the Regulations apply to persons appointed as Supervisors of Midwives on or after that date, but in view of the importance of entrusting this work to persons with the necessary qualifications and experience, the Minister suggests that each Authority should review their arrangements for the supervision of midwives and should take the earliest opportunity for effecting any changes which may be desirable having regard to the qualifications prescribed by the Regulations. This is of particular importance at the present time when the new service of salaried midwives under the Act of 1936 is about to be established throughout the country.

(3) The Departmental Committee on Midwives, which reported in 1929, pointed out that the inspection of midwives by a person without adequate experience of practical midwifery has a bad psychological effect upon the midwife and reacts unfavourably on her methods of practice, as she is deprived of the opportunity for guidance on professional matters affecting the well-being of her patients which she would receive from a property qualified inspector. In particular, the Committee strongly deprecated

the employment as inspectors of midwives of Health Visitors with little or no practical experience of midwifery. The Minister endorses these views and it will be seen that the Regulations require that persons appointed in future to supervise midwives shall have had adequate experience in the practice of midwifery.

(4) The Departmental Committee also drew attention to the fact that an inspector of midwives should be regarded as the counsellor and friend of the midwives, rather than a relentless critic and should be one who is ready to instruct the midwives in the various points of difficulty which arise from time to time in connection with their work and make them feel that there is always someone to whom they can look for sympathetic understanding of the laborious nature of their profession. The Minister feels that it is scarcely necessary for him to emphasize the importance of appointing persons who not only possess the necessary professional qualifications, but who also have the essential qualities of sympathy and tact, and he thinks it desirable that the title of 'Inspector of Midwives' should be superseded by that of 'Supervisor of Midwives' which is that used in the Regulations.

(5) The Regulations prescribe qualifications for a Medical Supervisor, and a non-Medical Supervisor, respectively, and it is within the discretion of each Authority to appoint either one or the other, or both. But in large areas it appears to the Minister that the most desirable arrangement would generally be to appoint a Medical Supervisor, acting under the direction of the Medical Officer of Health, to exercise general supervision over the midwives practising in the area, and non-Medical Supervisors to work under the instructions of the Medical Supervisor and perform the routine duties of supervision.

(6) The Minister appreciates that at the outset it may be difficult in some cases to secure Medical Supervisors who possess all the qualifications prescribed in Article 3 of the Regulations, and if necessary he will be prepared to consider the question of using dispensing power which is contained in Article 5. He thinks it desirable, however, to point out that the words 'some branch of obstetric work' in Article 3 have a wide range, and include the conduct of antenatal clinics, the duties of administrative officers in a maternity department, the investigation or treatment of puerperal fever, obstetric research, etc.

(7) In conclusion, the Minister wished to emphasize the fact that the duties of a Supervisor of Midwives extend to all the midwives practising in the area of the Authority and that a distinction should be drawn between an officer holding this post and one who is appointed as a Superintendent or Senior Midwife to control the work of the salaried midwives appointed by the Authority. The Minister is advised that it is not desirable for a Supervisor of Midwives to be engaged in the actual practice of midwifery.

(8) A copy of this circular has been sent to the Medical Officer of Health.

> I am, Sir,
> Your obedient Servant,
>
> Assistant Secretary.

In 1937 The Institute of Inspectors became the *Association of Supervisors.*

The 1951 Midwives Act laid a duty on Local Supervising Authorities to ensure that midwives attended Statutory Post graduate courses. The Supervisor of Midwives was requested to draw up the list of midwives who were due for attendance. This duty continues today.

The 1974 National Health Service (Re-organization) Act abolished the Local Supervising Authorities in their previous form and nominated Regional Health Authorities as Local Supervising Authorities. They delegated various duties to locally designated Supervisors of Midwives approved by the Local Supervising Authorities and nominated by the District Health Authorities.

The Midwives (Qualifications of Supervisors) Regulations 1977 No. 1580
These regulations gave the qualifications and experience required to become a Supervisor. They specified that Supervisors must undertake an Induction course. They eradicated the role of the Medical Supervisor and removed the words 'non-medical' from the title.

In 1978 the Central Midwives Board introduced courses of instruction for Supervisors, initially for those Supervisors new to a supervision post since 1974, but later they became mandatory for all Supervisors before or after appointment. (Rule 44 (2), Midwives Rules, 1986).

The 1979 Nurses, Midwives and Health Visitors Act abolished previous statutory bodies, created United Kingdom Central Council and National Boards, dividing the functions between them, but retaining Supervision of Midwives in *Sections 15 and 16*. Midwifery Committees are appointed to advise each body and comprise of elected and nominated professionals. Consultation with Midwifery Committees is mandatory on 'all matters related to midwifery' but there is no definition of what constitutes such matters except for the making or amending of rules of practice. All else therefore only requires consultation.

1980 – The Central Midwives Board issued its final Rule Book.

1983 – The Central Midwives Board issued its final Code of Practice.

1983 – The Central Midwives Board handed over to the new statutory body, the United Kingdom Central Council for Nurses, Midwives and Health Visitors.

1992 – Nurses, Midwives and Health Visitors Act made the UKCC the elected statutory body. The ENB continues with a midwife member but without a Midwifery Committee.

1994 – Midwives Code of Practice reworded the section on supervision to put less emphasis upon the control of midwives and more upon the partnership between midwife and supervisor.

(Compiled from ASM, 1992, Jenkins, 1995, Leap and Hunter, 1993 and RCM, 1988.)

What supervisors do

- be responsible for collection and collation of the midwives' intention to practise notices;
- conduct regular supervisory visits to each midwife to review her standard of practice, audit her drugs record and general record keeping and inspect her practice premises where necessary;
- advise the LSA in situations where there may be professional misconduct and where suspension from practice and referral to the UKCC is being considered;
- assess the training needs of the midwives she supervises, identify new skills for which training is required, facilitate any such training and ensure that all midwives have the opportunity to meet the requirements for refresher courses;
- provide supply order forms for the supply of pethidine and act as an authorized person for the destruction of controlled drugs (this is rarely required);
- be available to the midwives she supervises to discuss practice issues (the Code of Practice particularly highlights the need for the supervisor to be available if a midwife fails to obtain medical support for a home confinement or where the parents refuse medical cover);
- receive notifications of maternal deaths, stillbirth or neonatal death from midwives and, where necessary, investigate the circumstances of the death; and
- arrange for the medical examination of a midwife if it is thought necessary to prevent the spread of infection.

(Jenkins, 1995).

Local Supervising Authority and The Midwife

Kate Harmond

Regional Midwife, NHS Executive, North Thames RHA

Introduction

This paper aims to provide information about midwifery supervision and the way it is managed within North Thames. There is a wealth of literature describing the statutory responsibilities and supporting framework for midwives. This paper provides a brief overview for interested parties and explains the local approach to supervision.

North Thames Regional Health Authority

North Health Regional Health Authority (RHA) was formed in April 1994 from the previous North East and North West Thames RHAs. The RHA includes inner-city, suburban and rural populations, with a wide range of ethnic and social groups, all of which have particular needs and priorities. The RHA retains, among other functions, statutory responsibility for the supervision of midwives.

The RHA will be working in parallel to the Regional Office of the NHS Executive until April 1996.

The Local Supervising Authority for midwives

The Local Supervising Authority (LSA) for midwives will remain located at RHA level until April 1996.

The LSA is responsible for ensuring that supervision of midwifery practice is exercised to a satisfactory standard within its geographical boundaries.

This statutory responsibility applies to hospital and community midwives employed in the NHS, the private sector, prisons, those engaged in independent practice and those employed by general practitioners.

All practising midwives must notify the LSA of their intention to practice by 31 March each year using the form supplied by the United Kingdom Central Council for Nursing, Midwifery and Health Visiting (UKCC).

Functions of the LSA

The LSA is responsible for *appointing supervisors* of midwives and for providing a framework for supporting the supervision of midwifery practice within the region.

The LSA has a system for ensuring that each midwife is *eligible to practice* and for notifying this to the UKCC.

The LSA is responsible for ensuring that supervisors have access to initial and follow-up *education and training* and leads the development of standards and audit of supervision.

The LSA manages *communications* with supervisors of midwives, including the distribution of relevant NHS Executive Letters, hazard notices and other central documents and holds regular meetings to support supervisors and to develop key areas of practice.

The LSA has the authority to *suspend from practice* any midwife who has contravened the Midwives' Rules and/or Code of Professional Conduct, or Code of Practice, and who is felt to have acted in an unsafe or negligent manner, regardless of outcome to mother or baby.

Structure of North Thames LSA

The responsible regional officer in North Thames is Mrs Kate Harmond. (Telephone number 0171 725 5492, Facsimile Number: 0171 402 5207)

There are six link supervisors within North Thames Region who have specific responsibilities:

- To help investigate alleged professional misconduct or associated untoward incidents.
- To lead or participate in national initiatives e.g. Confidential Enquiries, education and practice projects, English National Board Projects.
- To act as a resource for other supervisors and the LSA.

Process

The LSA meets every three to four months with all Heads of midwifery, with other supervisors invited to attend or deputize and at least annually with all supervisors for updating and education purposes. These meetings may lead to the development of working groups to address issues of concern by publishing guidance e.g. on mental health in pregnancy.

In addition, the LSA arranges workshops and seminars for supervisors on topics relating to professional practice.

The LSA will act as external assessor where requested for appointment of new supervisors and offers individual orientation meetings.

The LSA is a point of referral for telephone and written enquiries and can offer informal and formal advice on issues relating to supervision.

The LSA will also investigate untoward incidents and complaints if requested by a Trust or Health Authority.

The LSA and link supervisors maintain contact with national developments by twice yearly meetings with the English National Board.

Role of the supervisor

While the appointment of a supervisor of midwives is the responsibility of the LSA these appointments are normally made on the recommendation of the Head of Midwifery Services (or equivalent) within the Trust.

A minimum requirement is that the supervisor is eligible to meet national criteria published by the UKCC, and that she or he has successfully completed the recognized course for the preparation of supervisors approved by the ENB.

Selection of supervisors should not automatically be attached to a 'post', whether managerial or educational, but should take into consideration the individual's wishes, capacity and potential.

The LSA supports the selection of new supervisors by means of internal advertisement and competitive interview and may assist in this process on request.

Grading of supervisors

There is no compulsory correlation between the grade of the post and the potential to be a supervisor of midwifery, providing that the minimum national criteria are met.

The grading of any appointment is at the discretion of the Trust and supervisors may be on clinical grading, a nursing or senior management spine or in an educational grading structure.

Developmental posts for supervisors

The LSA encourages a flexible approach to ensuring effective supervision to meet local needs and welcomes the development of creative packages to meet these needs. There is no objection to new or potential supervisors 'shadowing' more experienced colleagues for an agreed period of time, either within or outside the employing Trust, provided that confidentially is assured.

The LSA supports the creation of supervisors' posts which may be combined with a research, audit or development role, thus improving the risk assessment potential within the Trust.

Team leaders and supervision

As maternity care is increasingly arranged within semi-autonomous teams of mid-wives, the LSA would support the team leaders being trained as supervisors.

An effective model might involve these team leaders supervising the midwives of another team, while perhaps a midwife educationalist supervisor might supervise all the team leaders. This model would also help reinforce the differences between management and supervisory responsibilities.

Non managerial supervisors

The LSA strongly recommends that all supervisors should hold a caseload of practising midwives for whom they do not have direct line management responsibility. Supervisors do not need to be in clinical management posts to fulfil this recommendation: for example the senior midwife in the Trust may supervise independent, agency and educationalist midwives, while senior midwife educationalists may supervise the midwives in neonatal and fertility services.

The LSA will only appoint supervisors who are direct employees of the NHS, or whose clinical practice is concentrated almost wholly to the NHS. This is because of the clear organizational relationships e.g. between Trusts, Commissioning Authorities and the LSA, and their common regulatory framework.

Continuing education

The ENB has recently published changes to the continuing educational requirements for supervisors. The LSA in North Thames will support the implementation of these changes by making appropriate arrangements for updating supervisors who trained under the 'old' system.

These changes do not detract from individual midwives' responsibilities to retain and attain professional competencies.

Deselection of supervisors

The LSA has the capacity to remove supervisory status under exceptional circumstances and has taken such steps where necessary. Criteria for deselection include substantiated cases of misconduct or negligence, on request of the individual supervisor, reasons of ill health or personal and confidential reasons.

It may be useful to note that such deselection is rare, but these decisions have usually been received with relief by the supervisor concerned. All cases are, where possible, discussed individually with the supervisor and a representative of her or his choice.

Supervisors and the private sector

Supervisors also have responsibility for non-NHS midwives, including those in independent practice and those employed by agencies, general practitioners or private hospitals. The LSA recognizes that for reasons of geography some supervisors have a disproportionate responsibility for non-NHS midwives – for example where there are large private maternity hospitals, or other non-NHS institutions such as women's prisons, special hostels or psychiatric nursing homes with mother and baby units.

The LSA supports the principle of payment to the Trust for input from these supervisors for duties over and above their statutory responsibilities.

Good inter-institutional relationships can be mutually rewarding with opportunities for joint training, external clinical placements/experience and shared policy or practice developments.

On call arrangements
Arrangements for access to a supervisor of midwives are the responsibility of the local Trust.

Each trust has a different approach and philosophy, ranging from 24 hour on site cover by supervisors to informal non-rostered availability. Most 'out of hours' crises can be dealt with by the responsible manager in the immediate instance, but the supervisors may be needed to support staff and provide leadership when an untoward incident has occurred. If informal systems for access to the supervisor are acceptable to the Trust, it must be clear to all staff that it may not always be possible to contact one of 'their' supervisors at any particular time.

Cross cover arrangements
Supervisors are appointed to a District Health Authority not a Trust and have responsibilities beyond their employment boundaries, which can be included in their job descriptions.

The LSA encourages the use of cross District boundary cover between supervisors to compensate for absences or to facilitate rostering arrangements.

Supervisors are frequently asked to provide expert external advice to Trusts or other organizations: if this involves a whole day or more, it is reasonable for the supervisor's employer to charge for such services. The LSA does not advise on the amount of such charges, which may not normally be paid to the individual supervisor.

It may be useful for supervision requirements to be made explicit in maternity contracts with purchasers.

Standards for supervision
1. Each supervisor will have a caseload of named midwives preferably those for whom they do not have direct line management responsibility.
2. Each supervisor will have a caseload of between five (minimum) and thirty (maximum) named midwives.
3. Each supervisor will hold formal and individual meetings at least once a year with those midwives to review educational, training, practice and development needs.
4. Each supervisor will ensure that arrangements for refresher in advance so that individual learning can be addressed.

5. Each supervisor will ensure that midwives give formal feedback, either orally or in writing, after any training or educational activity funded by the Trust.
6. Each supervisor will hold a package of information and documents which will be available to the midwives for reference at any time.
7. Each supervisor will produce an annual report for the LSA using the agreed format.

The supervisor should be aware of all midwives practising within the boundaries of the local health authority. Where there is more than one maternity unit within a health authority's boundaries, the LSA should ensure there is agreement about the geographical area covered by each unit for the purposes of supervision.

The supervisor is concerned with the standards of practice of all midwives including their work, records and equipment, regardless of their place of employment.

Professional misconduct

Allegations of professional misconduct should in the first instance be investigated by the local unit and a suggested format for reporting such incidents to the LSA is available. It is recommended that the LSA is informed by telephone as soon as possible after any untoward incident.

All cases referred to the LSA in North Thames are presented· to the Regional Officer together with a 'link' supervisor who has not been involved in the initial investigation. This presentation is normally undertaken by the local 'investigating' supervisor.

Analysis of this presentation may lead to the suspension from practice of a midwife who has contravened the Midwives Rules and/or Code of Professional Conduct, or Code of Practice and who is felt to have acted in an unsafe or negligent manner, regardless of outcome to mother or baby.

The analysis may also result in the referral of the midwife to the Preliminary Proceedings Committee of the UKCC, without suspension from practice or to no action being taken. It is also possible that a referral to the UKCC health commitee may be made.

The LSA is responsible for supplying all the necessary written communications in these cases.

Supervised practice

The LSA may request that a supervisor arranges a period of supervised practice for a midwife from another unit if so directed by the UKCC. In these cases, the midwife should be given supernumary status, an honorary contract and an agreed set of learning objectives.

Providers and supervision

General Practitioners: GPs may employ practice nurses who are also practising midwives. The midwives must notify their intention to practise to a local supervisor (normally at the nearest NHS hospital) if they intend to practise as a midwife.

GPs may not allow non-practising midwives to undertake midwifery care, such as antenatal, postnatal or intra partum care. Nurses who undertake midwifery duties may find themselves liable to investigation for professional misconduct.

Hospitals and Community Trusts: There may be problems in obtaining consensus about managerial and supervisory responsibilities when an untoward incident occurs. The LSA provides a format to help supervisors decide on appropriate action.

If the midwife's professional conduct is an issue of concern, it is essential that the employing authority obtains appropriate supervisory advice, in the first instance from the local supervisor in the Trust. The supervisor should undertake the initial investigation, liaising as necessary with the LSA, where the responsible officer can offer guidance and support. It should be noted that local management policies cannot be allowed to override the midwife's professional codes of practice, conduct and rules; and that supervisors have a duty to support midwives who act within their professional sphere of practice and common law.

Independent midwives: Self-employed midwives in private practice should have access to a named supervisor in the local NHS unit. It is recommended that supervisors accept a standard equipment checklist certificate to avoid duplication of effort.

Individual Trusts should have available policies relating to independent midwives. Supervisors should note the necessity to ensure that:

- the midwife is eligible to practice.
- that arrangements for emergency care are agreed.
- that an honorary contract is available if the midwife is to practice on NHS premises.
- that effective communications systems involving the midwife, her client, medical staff and the supervisor are established between all parties.
- that liability insurance issues are agreed between the midwife and the Trust

Private sector

Supervisors are responsible for ensuring acceptable standards of midwifery care in the private sector as well as the NHS and should visit such local units regularly to provide advice and guidance.

This may include offering updating and education opportunities to these midwives, investigating and reporting to the LSA any untoward incidents and ensuring a regular system of communications with visits and telephone contacts.

North Thames LSA does not appoint supervisors of midwives outside the NHS.

Commissioners and supervision

Changing Childbirth

EL 94/9 sets out the responsibilities of commissioning authorities to achieve the recommendations of 'Changing Childbirth'; it may be helpful for commissioners to access the expertise of supervisors to support this.

Maternity Services Liaison Committees

Commissioning authorities may wish to include local supervisors on these committees to help progress developments and advise on changes in midwifery care.

LSA responsibilities

The functions and manpower review (1994) resulted in the planned abolition of RHAs in 1996: it is probable that the new health authorities will take on additional responsibilities for supervision in the future. An options appraisal exercise is underway between the LSA and commissioners within North Thames to explore the best way for taking this forward.

Glossary of Terms

Head of Midwifery	The senior midwife responsible for the organization of hospital and community midwifery services.
Trusts	Includes NHS hospitals which are still directly managed units or Special Health Authorities.
She	Can be substituted by 'he' where appropriate
Commissioners	Also known as purchasers or purchasing authorities

Where Supervision Goes Wrong

Breda Seaman
RM, RN

Introduction

The problems I meet in my daily work mainly arise from the inability to provide choice, control and continuity of care to the women I care for. I have also faced the threat of downgrading, (I am fortunate to be a G grade midwife, one of an endangered species) and seem to possess a fatal attraction to disciplinary action in the last two years.

There is one specific problem within my field of practice which hinders the effective provision of a good service to the women. It saddens me to acknowledge that the single overriding issue which causes me to want to leave the midwifery profession today, if it were financially feasible for me to do so, is the negative experience I have had of midwifery supervision.

The two strange cases of triple supervision
Case one
I am unable to disclose details of the initial case due to confidentiality and on going inquiries. However the manner in which the supervisory aspects of the case were dealt with is the subject for discussion.

I was requested to attend a meeting with my supervisor of midwives, and the contact supervisor. Two hours prior to the meeting I was informed that the Link supervisor would also be present. I became suspicious when the unit general manager telephoned, notifying my midwifery manager/supervisor of midwives that a friend or trade union representative could accompany me to the meeting. *I was not aware that this was necessary for a supervisory meeting.*

I informed my manager that I was *unhappy to attend the meeting* as there was insufficient notice to get a union official. However I was informed that I could not refuse to attend *a supervisory meeting* and told 'not to be so paranoid'. I was also surprised that my own supervisor who was at that stage my line manager was not actively involved in the meeting although she sat in on for the duration without saying a word. (I was later informed that she was there in a learning capacity).

Following the meeting I received a letter which stated that; 'through your actions you failed to provide appropriate midwifery care and had breached the UKCC Code of Professional Conduct particularly section 2.2.7 and the UKCC Midwife's Code of Practice, section 3.5 (rule 42).'

I remain to this day utterly puzzled regarding the first charge, as section 2.2.7 does not exist in the Code of Professional Conduct. It is cited in the UKCC Midwife's Code of Practice. I appreciate that the Code of Professional Conduct is distinct from but complementary to the Code of Practice and that supervisors of midwives are only human and subject to error. My cynical nature leads me to believe that if questioned I would be informed that it was due to a typing error.

My standard of midwifery practice was found to be unsatisfactory and although *formal Local Supervising Authority action was not recommended* my midwifery practice was to be assessed and a programme of professional development planned and implemented.

I was horrified when I received a letter two weeks later requesting me to attend a meeting following *investigations* into the standard of my midwifery practice. The *supervisory* meeting I had attended was now termed an *investigative one*. I was notified that as the outcome may result in disciplinary action I may be accompanied by an accredited representative of a staff organization, or by a friend not acting in a professional capacity.

The following week I received another letter informing me that a decision had been reached to implement the disciplinary procedure. I was requested to attend in three weeks. However I was becoming rather uneasy about the fact that the Director of Midwifery who had by default become my supervisor, and who initially interviewed/investigated me was to be on the disciplinary panel. I believe this was bad practice but one of many examples that followed! Representation was provided by the Royal College of Midwives, Industrial Relations Department. This 'supervisor of midwives' was replaced at the request of my representative.

The outcome was that I was issued with a first Written Warning to remain on file for one year. (It actually was on file for 15 months despite repeated verbal requests for written confirmation of removal. There appeared to be a perverse sense of joy from the 'supervisor' in prolonging the duration of the warning).

The conditions attached to the warning included:

1. A full assessment of current levels of competence.
2. Evidence of updating is required to be provided and a training programme implemented.
3. Evidence will be required to show that policies and procedures of the unit are carried out.
4. Assessment of the above will be undertaken in three months to determine that improvement has occurred.

I was also advised that if there was no improvement during the three month period, or if it was found that I have not co-operated fully with the conditions, then further disciplinary action could be taken.

My instant reaction was to appeal. I liaised with the industrial relations officer. The advice I received was;

The Manager who gave the written warning is not herself a midwife. She therefore relied on the advice she received from a Midwifery Manager; (the one who was informed that she could not sit on the panel) as well as the view expressed by the Local Supervising Authority. Any appeal panel is likely to comprise of people who are not midwives. Therefore they will have to rely on the same advice. The greater likelihood is that, given the need to make a choice, the appeals panel will come down on the side of management. Furthermore, there is always the outside possibility that any re-examination could lead to a reference to the UKCC.

In a nutshell I was in a catch 22 position. The system offers no justice to midwives. The Director was now assuming all pervasive powers in all matters relating to the unit and *for the next ten months I had no named Supervisor of Midwives.*

In essence I was committed to keeping a low profile for a year. A difficult task for an enthusiastic innovative midwife. I also lived with the underlying anxiety of possible referral to the UKCC as the midwifery supervisor made reference to this on numerous occasions. *As midwifery management were in liaison with the Royal College of Midwives I wondered on many occasions who really was the RCM supporting? Grassroots midwives or Midwifery Management?*

Three months later I received another letter setting out the action required of me in accordance with the decisions taken at the disciplinary hearing and the letter received from the Local Supervising Authority. I was to be seconded from my base of employment to the Consultant Unit for period of two months minimum.

I then received another letter from my manager requesting me to attend her 'office' to discuss an alleged incident which was not pursued and proved to be a further effort to intimidate me. By this stage I was convinced that I was being subject to harassment and victimization. However I maintained some form of sanity, undertook my two month programme of professional development and made every effort to fully comply with the management's instructions.

At no time did I receive any guidance, friendship or counselling from any supervisor of midwives.

Whilst at the Consultant unit my support came from the student midwives and newly qualified midwives who seemed impressed at my ability to empower women in a high tech unit to achieve a normal birth. At the Consultant unit the women who I cared for achieved 70 per cent normal births. However I must admit I failed to gain competence in suturing episiotomies, basically because I do not routinely perform them. The time went by very quickly and I was relieved to leave the Consultant unit and return to base. On my re-appearance at my work base some local women enquired as to the disappearance of 'their named midwife' for the past two months as they had received no explanation of my absence.

I submitted an evaluation of my experience, but did not receive any feedback from any manager /supervisor /educationalist.

Whenever I communicated with the supervisor of midwives there was always an element of threats emerging from her e.g. I should admit to an error of judgement in respect of the case and everything would be all right.

The pressure to keep a low profile was very intense.

I found the work environment extremely stressful and one morning some six months after these events started I suffered an asthmatic attack due to stress and pressure. I had no previous history of asthma.

Case two

Some ten months following the disciplinary hearing I wanted to take a grievance out against the Director of Midwifery Services due to persistent victimization and harassment. I was advised by the Royal College of Midwives not to. Throughout a period of 16 months there was no element of caring for the carers. The heavy policing of midwifery was very evident.

The 'Heathrow Debate' (1993) discussed the challenges for nursing and midwifery in the 21st century, and addressed the issues of supervision and accountability. Contributors recommended that,

> 'What is meant by supervision will require careful reassessment. It should not be policing, but should be a framework to support autonomous, professional performance, involving agreed aims and peer review.'

I had a period of five months free from a disciplinary on my record.

Then in December 1994 I had a disagreement with a colleague regarding the management of a woman. I sought the assistance of the midwifery supervisor, someone who was now separate from my line management. I was advised by my supervisor to complete an incident form and submit it to my manager, so that she could deal with the matter and resolve it locally.

Naturally I took the advice given to me by my supervisor. The result was that my manage did not seek to resolve the matter and establish the facts of the case relating to why there had been a professional disagreement about the management of the case. Rather I was asked to attend a meeting along with my colleagues which the clinical director convened.

Flint, (1988) states that,

> 'the UK seems to be the only country where midwives are at threat from members of their own profession, the only country where midwives use as a primary recourse the disciplinary system when trying to deal with practitioners who are strong, enthusiastic and outspoken.'

Each midwife was allocated a ten minute appointment. The midwifery manager stated that she was unaware of the contents of the meeting. It was generally perceived that we would be informed about clinical regrading.

However it soon transpired that supervision of midwifery was now being dealt with by the higher echelons of the clinical directorate. No fewer than five senior managers were present, of which three were supervisors of midwives, a most intimidating and harrowing experience.

I was questioned about my practice in regard to the case but more serious were the personal accusations made against me. They included the suggestion that my colleagues would not work with me and that the Clinical director had in his possession written complaints against me. He refused to substantiate any of these accusations with actual evidence.

Following this meeting I now find myself with another first written warning to be placed on file for a period of 24 months. I am currently in the process of appealing and have been advised not to partake in this conference. However as a innovator and change agent I accept that I will be hated and hounded. What is unfortunate though this will be undertaken by members of the midwifery profession.

Lessons to be learnt

I whole heartedly agree with Lansdell, (1989) who wrote,

> 'The relationship between supervisor and midwife is a very special one. It must be based on mutual trust and respect, and needs to be nurtured if it is to be of maximum benefit to the individual midwife.'

However, the local information pack on midwifery supervision, states that:

> Previously a reactive approach meant that we only appeared to act once a midwife had problems identified with her practice. It is the hope of all the local Supervisors that a new proactive approach to supervision will ensure that all midwives are prepared and supported for their future role, as described in 'Changing Childbirth'. (Department of Health,1993)

Is blatant victimization, harassment and managerial confusion, the evidence of the new proactive approach to midwifery supervision?

If it is the future is very bleak for the midwifery profession.

Role of supervisor of midwives, is it necessary?

Supervision is the monitoring of standards of practice as outlined in the Midwives Rules and Code of Practice and the monitoring of the practice of all midwives working within an area. It is a statutory responsibility undertaken to protect the public and support the midwife. Flint (1988) highlights the need to address the role of the supervisor of midwives as harassment of midwives increases.

Is the role of the supervisor of midwives really helpful? Can the role of the supervisor who initiates allegations of professional misconduct also provide friendship, guidance and counselling?

It is always difficult defining supervision as opposed to management. There are many, often conflicting, definitions of supervision. Thus, in the social work field, Ford and Jones (1987) view it as:

> 'planned regular periods of time that supervisor and supervisee spend together discussing the (students) work in the placement and reviewing the learning process.'

Brammer and Wassmer (1977) in the training of counsellors regard supervision as the assignment of an experienced person to help a beginner through the use of case material. To nurses, however, supervision means something quite different. It is usually associated with 'observation by an administrative superior who inspects, directs, controls and evaluates the nurses work' and often has negative connotations (Platt-Koch 1986).

All these professionals have two professional relationships – their relationship with their client and their relationship with their professional body. However, midwifery has an extra relationship which is with the supervisor of midwives, which is a statutory requirement within the Nurses, Midwives and Health Visitors Act of 1979, amended in 1992. The Act serves 'to regulate and restrict within due limits the practice of midwives and to protect the public from unsafe practitioners'. The supervisor's role is, or should be, administratively, structurally and, in some ways, morally, distinct from her role as manager of the maternity services, notwithstanding the fact that she frequently carries out both sets of duties. Walking on this path of conflicting interests could be a reason why an increasing number of midwives are finding themselves in difficult and vulnerable positions due to the clouding of issues between midwifery supervision and managerial policies. However, Landsell (1989) argues that it is preferable to combine these two roles, if only because the problems which the counsellor and friend needs to solve require the authority of managerial action.

However, all too frequently supervisors of midwives get enmeshed in managerial issues so that the guide, friend and counsellor aspects receive minimal, if any, consideration. It is a sad reflection on midwifery supervision that midwives cannot be empowered and supported in their work, in the same way that they are expected to support and empower the mother.

Historically the words 'See Me In My Office', ARM (1984) alerted midwives to potential problems. Many responded in total innocence, not realizing that when they emerged from the office they had to face up and cope with the drastic consequences, usually on their own. This occurs because the guide, friend and counsellor role of the supervisor of midwives is frequently absent at these traumatic times. Clearly there is a pressing need to resolve this role confusion, particularly the conflict between the supervisor as investigator of alleged misconduct or malpractice and as emotional supporter.

In the ever changing climate of the National Health Service the role of the Supervisor of Midwives has become a bouquet of barbed wire. In fact one Regional Health Authority disregarded the important role of the Local Supervising Authority when the holder of the pot was made redundant. A gaping hole was left in the supervisory structure due to this error. Many Unit General managers and clinical directors are totally unaware of the role of the supervisor and have implemented disciplinary action following supervisory interviews. All too often supervisory interviews are suddenly termed 'investigative' interviews. *Management tends to tackle problems through accusation and presumption of guilt before establishing the full facts and sorting out underlying problems.* In my experience and in other cases of which many of us are aware the haste with which investigative/disciplinary meetings are called render it near impossible to obtain, inform and brief properly professional and trade union representation. The current demand for such assistance has placed a heavy burden on the resources of these organizations.

When an incident occurs today the midwife is not summoned to 'The Office', instead she is requested to complete an incident form or submit a statement of fact. The submission of these forms can further implicate the midwife. However, supervisors and managers constantly reassure midwives that the completion of the forms is in their own interest. Frequently midwives are then requested to amend their statements when the problem becomes a thorny issue for management. It is small wonder then that some midwives personal files are ever increasing in size.

Supervision is what makes us strong, helps us develop our practice, provides support and distinguishes us as a profession (Davis, 1994). At its best, supervision empowers the midwife. At the other extreme, bad supervision can destroy a caring midwife. It is not the principle of supervision that is under attack, but its operation.

The Role of The Supervisor of Midwives requires urgent reappraisal for the challenges of 'Changing Childbirth' (Department of Health, 1993) to be successfully implemented.

References

Brammer, L.M., Wasserman, A.C. (1977). 'Supervision in counselling and Psychotherapy'. In Kurpius, D.J. *Training.* Wewstport,Connecticut: Greenwood Press.

Davis, K. (1994). 'Is statutory supervision central to our professional identity?' *British Journal of Midwifery.* Vol 2, No 7.

Department of Health (1993) . *Changing Childbirth: The Report of the Expert Maternity Group.* London: HMSO.

Department of Health (1994). *The Challenges for Nursing and Midwifery in the 21st Century.*

Flint, C. (1988). 'On the brink, midwifery in britain' In Kitzinger, S. (Ed.) *The Midwife Challenge.* p.32

Flint, C. (1988). 'The Golden Thread', *Association of Radical Midwives Magazine* No 37, p.18–19.

Ford, K., Jones, A. (1987). *Student Supervision.* Basingstoke: MacMillan..

Landsell, M. (1989). 'Friend and Counsellor', *Nursing Times* 85 (28), p.86.

Platt-Koch, L.M. (1986). 'Clinical Supervision for psychiatric nurses'. *Journal of Psychological Nursing.* 26; 1; pp.7–15.

Wilde, C. (1984). 'See Me In My Office' *Association of Radical Midwives* No.23.

UKCC (1992a*). Code of Professional Conduct.*

UKCC (1994). *The Midwife's Code of Practice.*

Conflicts in Supervision of Midwives

Irene Walton

Supervision of midwives is a mechanism, laid down in statute, for ensuring that midwifery practice in the United Kingdom is of the highest standard. Its overall aim is to protect the public and ensure that the safety of mother and baby is paramount. This being so, it does not at first glance seem to hold the potential for conflict but in practice it throws up conflict at different levels and in different ways.

Supervision is laid down in the Nurses, Midwives and Health Visitors Acts of 1979 and 1992 under which provision is made to enable the United Kingdom Central Council (UKCC) to formulate rules regulating the practice of midwives which may in particular:

Section 15.- (1)
a) determine the circumstances by means of which, midwives may be suspended from practice;

b) require midwives to give notice of their intention to practice to the local supervising authority for the area in which they intend to practice; and

c) require registered midwives to attend courses of instruction in accordance with the rules.

Nurses, Midwives and Health Visitors Act 1979 (Section 15.[1]) p.11)

This section introduces an inspectorial or policing function which is implicit in the term 'supervision'. However in addition to the provision of rules under Section 15 there is the requirement under section 16 for general supervision of midwives by the Local Supervising Authority (LSA). (House of Commons 1979 Section 16.2.a).

Although much of the duty of the LSA is concerned with discharging its statutory functions of keeping records, investigating prima facie cases of misconduct and determining whether or not to suspend a midwife from practice, there is also an obligation (non statutory) to be a support for the midwife. This is clarified in the Midwife's Code of Practice (1994) and devolved to the supervisor of midwives:

51. Your supervisor of midwives should give you support as a colleague, counsellor and advisor. This should be developed in order to promote a positive working relationship which is conducive to maintaining and improving standards of practice and care. (UKCC, 1994)

The Supervisor of Midwives is thus left with the role of inspector on behalf of the LSA and that of a colleague. This will provide areas of conflict for her and for the midwives she supervises. As an inspector she must ensure that the midwife is working within the guidelines and policies laid down for safe practice. She must also satisfy herself that the midwife's record keeping complies with Rule 42 (UKCC, 1993) by periodically auditing the records. She will have to ensure that the midwife is keeping accurate records regarding controlled and prescription only drugs and that any discrepancies are investigated. Under Rule 43 she must inspect the 'practising midwife's methods of practice, her records, her equipment and such part of her residence that may be used for professional purposes' (UKCC, 1993 Section B. p.22). These duties of inspection must in some way distance the supervisor from the midwife being supervised. There is tremendous power inherent within the role and whilst most supervisors can cope with this and still remain a colleague to the midwives, others cannot. In reality some may even relish the control that such a role confers and become extremely authoritarian over the midwives who are being supervised. In this case power can be a dangerous thing and most certainly conflicts with the aim of enabling and facilitating midwifery practice.

Another aspect of conflict for the supervisor is that of her other 'hat'. Most supervisors are also managers and the role of the manager may overlap with that of supervisor. For example the manager aims to ensure that a high quality service is delivered to the public. This is totally consistent with the aim of a supervisor of midwives which is to ensure that midwifery care is delivered to a high standard. At first glance one would think that there could be no conflict in this because the aims are so alike. However it is in the achievement of the aims that there is a potential for conflict. The manager will achieve her/his aim through the mechanisms of job descriptions and individual performance review and staff employment issues. She or he will give support to the employee through equipment, the environment, administration and support systems, policies, procedures, protocols and appropriate skill mixes. The effectiveness of the midwife will be monitored against the job description and poor performance may result in disciplinary action which at worst could mean the midwife losing her/his job.

It is extremely difficult to separate this responsibility of a manager from that of a supervisor. The supervisor monitors the midwife's performance from a different aspect through annual review. She/he maintains a record of refresher courses and acquired and maintained competencies and aims to support the midwife by promoting good practice and facilitating communication channels, and ensuring that support services and appropriate mechanisms are in place e.g. general practitioner cover. She/he is there to facilitate the midwife in her practice and so should try to help the midwife to audit and evaluate her own practice and develop areas of perceived need. This may cause a supervisor/manager to be in conflict. She/he may find that a midwife admits to inadequacies in her role and as a manager may feel that the midwife should be downgraded to a more appropriate grade but as a supervisor she may find nothing wrong with the actual midwifery practice.

As a manager she/he will be an employee of a Provider Unit and will be committed to its mission statement and to its business plan. According to the ENB 'the aim of the manager is to achieve high quality service to meet contract specifications and make the best use of resources' (ENB, 1992). This may cause some conflict as a supervisor. For example, there may come a time when the labour ward is extremely busy and midwives have reported in sick. Although the Provider Unit has agreed to take women requiring admission, the Supervisor of midwives may deem that the conditions are not conducive to safe care. She/he must then make arrangements for further admissions to be taken by neighbouring Provider Units. She may find herself in some emotional turmoil as a result of this and will need the support of her supervisor colleagues. If she is not of sufficiently high level in the hierarchy she may feel very unsure of herself in a situation such as this.

Another cause of conflict to the Supervisor is the time commitment necessary to conduct supervision adequately and to act as a mentor to student supervisors. Although supervision is a statutory function and part of many a managers role it has not been timed or costed appropriately. This may result in it being conducted in a patchy, ad hoc fashion with some midwives being well supported whilst others may not have adequate support. This is particularly so when there are too few supervisors in post and each supervisor is supervising far more than the recommended 40 midwives each. As the requirement to be a supervisor of midwives is often part of the job description there is not usually a problem for midwifery managers within the NHS to actually act in the role. The problem is merely one of time management except (as anecdotal evidence suggests) where their manager is not a midwife and can see no difference between supervision and management. There is an argument that the Provider unit has to supply the elements contained in the role of the supervisor of midwives already as part of its quality assurance programme for the purchasers and so supervision is a luxury peculiar to midwifery.

There may be a problem of time commitment for midwives working outside the NHS. Midwifery education is now for the main part delivered from Colleges of Higher Education or Universities and midwife teachers who are Supervisors of midwives may find themselves on the horns of a dilemma. They may or may not get support from their establishment. Their work base may be far from the maternity unit and they may find the practicalities difficult because of distance. Midwives may also perceive the teacher-supervisor as being distanced in more ways than one and the closeness necessary for informal networking may no longer be there. Because there is no separately identified funding for supervision independent midwives as well as teachers who are not supported by their institution are precluded from becoming supervisors of midwives. This is a pity because not only does it prevent part of the profession from contributing and being part of the wider communications network but because some of the problems which cause conflict are due to the supervisor being also a manager. These would not be a problem if the supervisor was independent of the Provider Unit.

Policies and procedures may become an area of conflict for the supervisor as manager. In her/his capacity as a manager of the Provider Unit it is her/his duty to ensure that policies are both formulated and adhered to. These may be erring on the over cautious for many reasons e.g. the fear of litigation, and may reduce or negate the role of the midwife. Some policies which require certificates of competence to be signed by other health professionals work actively against the midwife's own responsibility and accountability under Rule 40 (UKCC, 1993). As policies are drawn up to maintain standards of safety, the issue of conflict here may be one of identifying and maintaining professional boundaries. There is also the problem that has been identified by Caroline Flint that in clinical practice there may be more than one way to care and 'midwifery suffers from a "nursing" model which says there is only one "right" way of doing things' (ARM, 1993). Trying to be both a conscientious employee and a promoter of midwifery practice may be problematic and give rise to the negativity that Caroline Flint (ARM, 1993) believes turns supervision into an oppressive tool.

This is particularly true when the supervisor has a problem with change management. One of the functions of the supervisor is to enable and facilitate the development of midwifery practice. The Midwives Rules are quite clear (Rule 40(2) UKCC 1993) that a midwife 'must not undertake any treatment which she has not been trained to give either before or after registration as a midwife'. If a midwife wants to develop a new care practice she must discuss it with her supervisor who will advise her on how to proceed. In the case of an innovation that is already in existence this may be in the form of helpful advice on gaining the necessary expertise and even a promise of being physically present to support the midwife in the early stages of the innovation. There may be a midwife who wants to do something which is so new that she cannot obtain training in this country before undertaking the procedure. Water birth came into this category in the beginning. The supervisor now has a problem. If she is experienced, knowledgeable and courageous she will assist the midwife to develop it as a research topic. This may mean ensuring the midwife undertakes a good literature search, discusses the theory and anticipates all the potential problems, has the informed consent and co-operation of the woman, and the necessary backup services. The supervisor will also ensure that she is present to help the midwife. This is endorsed by Jane Winship who emphasized at the UKCC working party that 'the use of legal power in professional practice is not about limiting practice but rather about legitimizing practice and enabling it to grow and develop' (Duff, 1994). Unfortunately innovation may cause a conflict for the supervisor as an employee and as a person if she cannot manage change. She will then retreat into the comfort of the status quo. This may impede development of care practices and will most certainly stifle innovation by the individual midwives. This issue caused Mavis Kirkham to pose the question as to whether midwives would be better supervised by their peers (Duff, 1994).

Managers may also have less time for clinical hands on care than they would like and as Professor Page pointed out 'it was more necessary than ever for supervisors to be in touch with midwives clinical dilemmas' (Duff, 1994). Sarah Roch also agreed that each supervisor should seek to achieve 'credibility in her role as a midwife' (Duff, 1994). This necessity to be clinically credible may cause conflict for the supervisor in that she may not have the time nor the inclination to maintain her clinical competency. It is also very difficult to maintain skills in all areas of practice without being somewhat vulnerable and this may not be something that managers wish to be. There is also the question of pseudo competence to consider. Taking a caseload of as few as four women a year cannot enable one to maintain clinical competency. For example there may only be one perineal laceration or episiotomy every two years which would hardly give the manager-supervisor the practice to remain proficient in suturing. Notable midwives including Meryl Thomas and Jane Winship have publicly stated that the midwife must be proficient in her area of practice which does not necessarily mean clinical hands on care. However, there is not universal agreement on this point and some supervisors insist on all the midwives they supervise including managers and teachers having clinical updates.

This shows up another area of conflict in supervision i.e. the lack of consistency and flexibility. Supervisors of midwives have a very good networking set up in the form of Regional supervisors meetings and can use these to disseminate information. They could also use these to ensure agreement on standards. This is particularly necessary now that the amendments in the 1992 Nurses, Midwives and Health Visitors Act Section 16.5 states 'that the Council may by rules prescribe standards to be observed with respect to advice and guidance'. If supervisors are pro-active in developing national standards for midwifery care this area of conflict may be reduced. This is more important than ever in the present climate of 'Changing Childbirth':

> 'One of the functions of the Supervisor is to maintain standards of midwifery care but before one can maintain a standard one must identify it and this is where effective supervision is helpful' and 'leading the work on the setting of standards will be the responsibility of the supervisor of midwives' (Walton and Hamilton 1995 p. 63-64).

The difficulty for some supervisors is that they misunderstand the difference between a standard which can state the required outcomes of good practice and a provider unit policy. This difficulty can result in out and out conflict when such a supervisor tries to use operational tools to supervise independent midwives. One of the hall marks of the profession is its practitioner status and this is clearly demonstrated by the existence of independent midwives. Good supervision supports and enables such midwives in their practice but where the supervisor is unclear about her role or is very controlling there will be difficulties not least of which will be for the childbearing woman concerned. In some areas there is now a slight movement towards peer review by the appointment of supervisors of midwives who are at F or G grade and this can either be a positive or a negative move. Positively it can move the profession towards a more equitable system of peer review where the supervisor can indeed be seen as a colleague, advisor and counsellor. But there are inherent negativities for the supervisor in that she may find it difficult to take on the appraisal, counselling and professional development aspects of the role with people who she works alongside every day. She may find it extremely uncomfortable to recommend another midwife's practice as poor and warranting investigation. This may not necessarily be an unsurmountable problem because as Meg Taylor (1994) points out although there may be problems of competitiveness, envy and a fear of assessment, if midwives were to receive training and skills in dealing with these problems a system similar to that in psychotherapy could evolve which would be both supportive and facilitative. Unfortunately it may evolve into the type of non statutory clinical supervision which is being considered for nurses and health visitors and which Karlene Davis fears may 'weaken midwives' arguments that they have ability to take on the lead role in providing woman centred care' (Davis, 1994). This would be a great pity because as Sarah Roch points out 'midwives must be clear of the strengths of Supervision and strive to make it work effectively' (Ferguson, 1994).

Another area of conflict for the lower graded supervisor of midwives is her lack of 'clout' in the Provider Unit hierarchy which may make her hesitant in putting forward controversial views. There may also be an inner conflict in that supervision issues may necessitate her moving away from Provider unit thinking and being human some supervisors may worry about their chances of future promotion. This would not be a problem if the selection procedure for supervisors clearly identified assertiveness as a criterion. The difficulty would be judging this in practice. However at this moment there are no clearly defined criteria for nomination and selection of prospective supervisors.

If the duality of the nature of supervision cause conflict for the supervisor of midwives it cause greater problems for the supervised midwife. The major problem as has been highlighted earlier is the inspectorial function. The possibility that the supervisor will find something inherently wrong with one's practice will inevitably lead the midwife to be wary. All midwives are concerned with the safety of mothers and babies and the vast majority are working with this aim in mind at all times. But midwifery care settings are undergoing such tremendous re-organizations and changes with midwives being required to take on board many innovations in a very short time. This coupled with a climate of redundancy and downgrading inevitably leads to stress. In the ideal supervisory situation the midwife should be able to turn to her supervisor for the support that she needs and many can in fact do so. The area of maximum conflict for the midwife is the issue of revealing problems to the supervisor. If there is to be open and honest communication between the two parties there should be the assurance of confidentiality. This would enable issues and dilemmas to be explored and the best solutions found. This is not possible where a midwife knows that if she either knowingly or unwittingly reveals a deficiency in knowledge or a potentially unsafe procedure she may have to be investigated with the worst scenario being removal from the register. It is not possible to treat the supervisor as a colleague, advisor and counsellor with the openness and trust that such a relationship requires if one is also likely to be disciplined and/or put on supervised practice by the same person. It is inevitable that a measure of wariness and suspicion will enter into the relationship. This is particularly so when the annual auditing process is used by an over controlling supervisor almost like a formal examination of competency. Revealing areas of practice where further development is needed may not always be a simple matter for the midwife. It may mean a period of update in another clinical area which could cause conflict with family arrangements. In this case there would be a temptation to minimize the need for such experience. It could also cause problems for the manager in the staffing arrangements.

More formal educational opportunities may be needed such as study days, refresher courses and even theoretical updating. Again this should not pose a problem if the end result is the personal and professional development of the midwife with the ultimate aim as an improvement in care. The conflict arises within the audit process itself where the assessment may not be a dialogue between equals but a form of judgement delivered by a superior. This is particularly so when there is an investigation interview following an incident of allegedly poor practice.

Midwives can find themselves brought before their supervisor (who may also be a manager in the provider unit) to answer questions on their practice. The incident may be very recent and if serious, the midwife could still be very shocked about it or it may be many months afterwards when memories may have faded. If the supervisor considers it necessary the midwife may be required to undergo supervised practice. There is no appeal system built into this procedure as Soo Down points out (ARM, 1993) which leads to a very unsatisfactory situation whereby midwives may justly feel very aggrieved and have no mechanism for redress.

The inspection process is firmly embedded in the statutory framework and in some ways conflicts with the role of a professional practitioner e.g. the inspection of bags and equipment. It seems rather strange to say the least that the content of a midwife's bag should be inspected by a supervisor. The practice does not seem congruous with the role of the midwife as an accountable practitioner who is capable of meeting the challenges of providing holistic midwifery care into the twenty first century. It certainly conflicts with the notion of the supervisor as a colleague and a peer.

Overall there are many conflicts inherent in supervision for midwives at all levels and although there is a section of the profession which would like to have it abolished altogether, there is another view which is that statutory supervision is a strength which should be developed and used as a powerful tool for the advancement of the profession and the continual safety of the mother and baby. This can only be done by reducing the inbuilt conflicts and cultivating supervision as an enabling mechanism for midwifery. In the first instance it would be helpful to completely separate out the inspectorial and administrative role from that of counsellor and colleague. This is the one major area from which conflicts arise and can be resolved practically by the inspectorial function being invested in a supervisor from another provider unit. The colleague aspect would be retained by the supervisor who works in the same provider unit as the midwife. If this is not thought to be possible the question must be posed as to why not. Is it a legal, ethical or business constraint? On first consideration it is probably the latter and if so ways must be found to overcome this hurdle. Criteria should be set for the nomination and selection of supervisors and there should be more specific counselling skills training given. Confidentiality should be assured from the supervisor who takes on the role of midwife supporter.

There should be an attempt to increase flexibility and to ensure consistency by national standard setting and developing supervision as a research based pro-active exponent of midwifery care. This could be linked to the wider approach to supervision e.g. computerization, where each midwife is supervised by one supervisor regardless of crossing boundaries.

It would be very useful if supervision was timed, costed and funded properly. If this was to happen there could be a more efficient system of safeguarding the public interest such as the 'Watchdog' scheme as envisaged by the Association of Radical Midwives (ARM, 1994). This could become part of the Purchaser's remit and would reduce a number of the conflicts described earlier and in particular that of being investigated by one's peer or colleague. It would also enable public involvement and a more democratic process which would give the midwife a right of appeal to an independent body.

Audit of supervision and the monitoring of supervisory performance against national standards and criteria would reduce the feeling of powerless that many midwives feel about supervision today. This coupled with a proper mechanism for deselection of supervisors would indeed enable the profession to develop. Supervision could become a mechanism for supporting midwives and enabling them to become innovative. They would have a safe environment in which to explore dilemmas of practice and truly identify their learning needs. If supervisors are to properly trained to take on their counselling role the midwife would also have a good support to explore feelings thrown up by experiences such as stillbirth or maternal death. Public safety would also continue to be safeguarded in a manner that did not automatically assume following a critical incident that the midwife was guilty of an offence, and misjudgment if it occurs would not necessarily be equated with misconduct.

References

Association of Radical Midwives (1993). 'Report of the Spring National Meeting' 20th March 1993 *Midwifery Matters* No. 57 Summer 1993 pp. 27–28.

Association of Radical Midwives (1994). 'Future Midwifery Supervision' *Midwifery Matters* No. 60 Spring 1994 pp. 25-27.

Davis, K.C. (1994). 'Is Statutory Supervision Central to Our Profes-sional Identity?' *British Journal Of Midwifery* Vol. 2 No. 7. July 1994 pp. 304–05.

English National Board (1992). *Preparation of Supervisors of Midwives: An Open Learning Programme* London: ENB.

Ferguson, P. (1994). 'RCM Annual Conference 1994 Report' *Midwives Chronicle and Nursing Notes* Vol. 107, No. 1280. p. 341.

Taylor, M. (1994). 'The Supervision of Midwives' *Midwifery Matters* No. 60 Spring 1995 p.28.

Duff, E. (1994), 'Meeting Report: UKCC Working Conference on Supervision of Midwifery' *Midwives Chronicle and Nursing Notes* Vol.107. No.1282. November 1994 pp.434-435.

House of Commons (1979). *Nurses, Midwives and Health Visitors Act* London: HMSO.

UKCC (1994). *A Midwife's Code of Practice.* May 1994 London: UKCC.

UKCC (1993). *Midwives Rules.* London: UKCC.

Walton, I., Hamilton, M. (1995). *Midwives and Changing Childbirth.* Hale: Books for Midwives Press.

Examples of Good Supervision

Jill Demilew

Background

During 1991 I interviewed 32 independent midwives (out of a possible 44) who had notified their intention to practice as 'independent' practitioners. This was nearly three quarters of midwives practising independently. Over a third had started independent practice within the previous two years.

The research was a sociological analysis of a 'crisis' within the British midwifery profession. Midwives are legislated to be autonomous practitioners yet their actual practice was severely limited in the NHS organizational structure. The reality was that midwives had semi-professional status and were midway in professional hierarchies and relatively powerless.

The interview schedule explored in depth:

1. What being a midwife and being a professional meant to the individual. It considered ideas of the professional/client relationship, of responsibility and accountability.
2. The midwife/supervisor relationship – it looked at the knowledge base of supervision and the individual's experience both whilst an NHS employee and during independent practice.
3. The relationships of the midwife with other health care professionals in institutional settings. This included midwives, obstetricians, paediatricians, GP's and Health Visitors. The practice of professional supervision and how it was experienced was analysed in great detail.
4. The future of midwifery practice and the maternity services in Britain.

The significance of research findings

I have chosen 'independent midwifery' because their ideology is the same as that which underpins the 'Changing Childbirth' government policy i.e.

1. 'that women should receive continuity of care during pregnancy and childbirth and a real choice in options for place of birth.'
2. Their chosen organization of midwifery care is a caseload model of practice.

Re-reading the research findings is uplifting because I realize how fast midwifery practice is changing and how far the profession has travelled towards *The Vision* (ARM, 1986). However, to proceed further, midwifery must address the fundamental question of the status of midwifery as a profession within the NHS and what this means for women and midwives.

Until this is faced, looking mechanically at supervision will merely be tinkering with an inappropriate tool. Supervision is just one particular method of professional regulation. The conference, however, may lead to *'Super-Vision'* by taking the midwifery profession forward towards building a system of professional regulation which is acknowledged, acceptable and truly accountable to women, midwives and medical colleagues and ultimately to our society.

Research findings – independent midwifery

Diane Martin (1990) looked at midwifery professional misconduct cases and concluded that midwives were damned if they did and damned if they didn't. She noted that midwives can be disciplined for not exercising accountability if they follow local policies or medical instructions blindly *or* they can be disciplined for exercising professional clinical judgement and not following locally accepted policies.

Knowledge base regarding supervision

84 per cent of the midwives said that they either couldn't remember or that the knowledge was insufficient for their practice.

Five midwives acknowledged that they had positive and good learning experiences from the role of supervisor. They made the proviso it was very different from how they observed supervision as practised. These five midwives had trained since 1987 during which time midwifery professional conduct received national media saturation during disciplinary cases e.g. Jilly Rosser and Chris Warren. Some tutors explored issues surrounding supervision very thoroughly. Notably four of these five midwives had tutors who were active members of ARM.

Supervisory experiences

All of the midwives powerfully articulated supervision being practised in a controlling, negative and obstructive way. They specifically noted that the result was to obstruct their clients from accessing the best quality care. This is a sad indictment. However two midwives spoke of their positive experiences of supervision. They felt,

'easy, informing them of every client, i.e. anything bordering on deviation from the norm as well as obvious deviation.'

'the supervision enabled the midwife to get the woman seen by an obstetrician.'

'able to get advice as well as support, and offered all the facilities available, i.e.

labour ward, day assessment unit, anything which works in the best interest of the client.'

Indeed they commented,

'this seems the way it should be going, to discuss anything without being censured for it.'

Ideology and supervision

There was a clear link between ideology and the practice of supervision and independent midwifery. If the midwife and supervisor had similar beliefs about the birth, professional practice and professional regulation then the relationship was positive and enabled women to access excellent quality care. If there were different belief systems then the potential and actual conflict was tense and potentially obstructive of appropriate care for women. Two out of the three of the midwives had had their professional practice investigated. One out of four had been investigated more than once. One in four had been investigated at the LSA level.

The future of supervision

The midwives had clear views as to how supervision, if retained, could be best practised to protect the public and enable them to practice autonomously, using their full role.

1. Advocacy for the midwife and woman – 75 per cent thought this to be a main function.
2. A third felt that the supervisors must enable a midwife to have access to hospital and facilities for clinical investigations.
3. A quarter made a plea to relate to one supervisor only whom they respected and had chosen.
4. A third of the midwives thought it inappropriate to have supervision at all in its current form.

Personal experiences

These mirror the research findings. Since the 'Winterton Report' and 'Changing Childbirth' have come a long way to legitimizing midwifery practice and making the profession more visible, life has become much easier. The best example of supervision has been solid support towards forging new systems and contracts within the NHS. The late Jeanette Brierly, Kate Jackson and Cathy Warwick (King's College Hospital, London) have supported the South East London Midwifery Group Practice to secure contracts with Health Commissioners for midwifery group practice in its own premises in the local community. Our other local provider units have equally given steady support in the light of considerable opposition from some other stakeholders in the maternity services.

Supervision – the future?

What are the key elements of good supervision that can be learned from this research?

What is the profession thinking about supervision?

What type of professional regulatory structure will meet the key aims of protecting the public and facilitating excellent professional practice?

Who will design it, building an acceptable, accessible and accountable system?

Any system of professional regulation in midwifery practice must:

1. Enable advocacy for women as individuals.
2. Enable advocacy for midwives as practitioners in the organization of the maternity services.
3. Enable clinical judgement within a setting of clinical excellence.

There was a resolution passed at the branch delegates meeting of the RCM at Annual Conference 1994 asking for a working party to be set up to look at the role of Supervisors of midwives. The aim is to strengthen the role of supervisors. The resolution specifically asked for particular areas to be considered:

a. selection of supervisors particularly possibility of local elections.
b. future role of supervisors and LSA's in the light of current and planned change in the NHS.
c. ensure appropriate expertise of Supervisors of midwives i.e. clinical competence and involvement.

Why are midwives asking for the role of supervision to be strengthened? They are clearly indicating their wishes for greater accountability and clinical credibility in those colleagues who become supervisors. They are equally aware that supervision needs to be re-examined in the light of organizational change. Until recent years supervision has been poorly taught, poorly understood and poorly practised. Whilst I recognize that beneficial changes are being made e.g. ENB Preparation Pack, and new directives from the Association of Supervisors about splitting the supervisory and managerial functions, there is a fundamental problem. My major concern is that supervision is not understood or accepted by many professional colleagues e.g. doctors and particularly by management in Trusts, Health Commissions and Regional Health Authorities. Supervision as a means to professional regulation is relatively powerless unless it is recognized, understood and accepted by all interested parties. If midwives, medical colleagues, employers and purchasers are hazy, misinformed or disillusioned about supervision what does it mean to the women whom we serve? Midwives want to control their practice and women would like an accountable service. From my research the positive supervisory experiences were concerned with accessing women to appropriate care i.e. consultation with obstetricians and choice of birth place attended by a midwife who they knew and trusted. This advocacy role should be needed when midwives are enabled to practice in all their local settings through a variety of contracts. Midwives should not need an intermediary to approach a consultant medical colleague or to direct an individual woman to appropriate care. Midwives should have direct access to the use of laboratory and ultrasound facilities and any facilities which enable them to practise midwifery fully and safely. This should be their right, not a privilege sanctioned through a supervisor or medical colleague.

The research also demonstrated that midwives wanted to be able to discuss their practice with someone who was approachable and easy to contact. They wanted this colleague to be someone who was clinically competent and able to understand the issues of clinical judgement in their sphere of practice. This professional consultation equally needs to be non-judgemental and confidential.

This research has demonstrated key areas which the midwifery practitioners perceive to be essential to excellent quality practice. Supervision in its current format is failing and far from being enabling, has been disabling with a few notable exceptions.

The status of the midwifery profession

This I believe to be the key component towards accountable excellent practice. Supervision has, until very recently, addressed its pro-active role very poorly. By this I mean that it has been perceived and experienced as a reactive and primarily disciplinary function or more worryingly as a nonentity and invisible. Issues relating to quality of service provision and enabling midwives to practice their role fully have been neglected e.g. staffing levels have been eroded, particularly in the postnatal areas. Clinical grading and professional pay continue to be chancrous sores to us in practice, with skill mix, re-profiling and local pay awards leading to hostility, apathy, distrust and frustration. Where is the leadership, who will take our profession forward? Supervision must first address these issues.

Action plan

1. The NHS Management Executive must address the employment structures and opportunities for midwifery practice. Midwifery is moving towards being a community based service firmly place with primary health care. However, midwives 'follow women' and practise in the hospital or acute care base as well. Caseload practice with midwives working together in small groups seems to be the appropriate model. Whether we label these groups, teams, partnerships or practices the central issue is for the midwives to be able to have control over their practice and be able to develop excellent quality, accountable and individualized care. Financial routes need to be worked out which acknowledge and facilitate these new systems of work. Medical and dental colleges have the option of being employed in hospitals in hierarchical models working shift systems *or* they can be self employed contracted in to the NHS in caseload models of practice. This demonstrates that different employment contracts and financial systems are appropriate for different models of practice. Midwives are not usually accepted as a separate profession from our nursing colleagues and certainly not an equivalent basis to medical and dental

colleagues. Midwifery needs to address the issue of equality of opportunity within the NHS. I make this plea because if we start from the basis, then from a firm foundation we can build an appropriate form of professional regulation.

2. We will continue tinkering with the current system to our peril. Clinical grading continues, local pay awards are on the horizon. There are divisions and disillusionment amongst midwives. A midwife may be expected to perform very differently for E, F and G grades depending on her differing job specifications in different areas in the country e.g. in one Trust if you are an E grade team midwife you are not allowed to perform a vaginal assessment on a woman labouring and planning to give birth at home. This is an obvious nonsense since it potentially doesn't meet that woman's need and is stopping that midwife from practising appropriately. Supervisors will be clear about this but what about the managers role and the implications for the midwifery budget?

3. The contract is very powerful and the purchasers have a responsibility to ensure that contracts require providers to have effective systems of audit. It can include issues of interprofessional working. Midwives need a workbase which they can own as theirs. It needs to be easily accessible to women locally. Current budgets have not been planned to take into account the costs of running a community based caseload model midwifery service. Maternity service contracts need to be drawn up to facilitate the different types of midwifery practice which will give women true choice and midwives choice in employment.

4. We are in an era of direct accountability. The 'Winterton Report' and 'Changing Childbirth' have forged forward because of the alliance of birthing women and midwives together. I propose that together, women and midwives, work towards an effective, acceptable and accountable system of professional regulation. It does not mean that we will discount the good elements of the current system of supervision. It frees the profession to build a strong foundation for an accountable, excellent quality midwifery service: a maternity service which fosters mutual respect between the professionals, but first and foremost the individual pregnant woman is the central focus.

Summary

I would endorse commitment towards:

1. Equal opportunities in employment in the NHS to facilitate the appropriate structural changes for providing an excellent quality midwifery service.
2. To build a new system of professional regulation together with organizations such as Maternity Alliance, AIMS and NCT.

Midwives are committed and willing to take the responsibility of professional practice. They require the right to be able to practice in the NHS. *Super-Vision* is the vision required to stop tinkering with a system that has singularly failed midwifery practice and build a solid foundation which will meet the challenge of 'Changing Childbirth' and the twenty first century.

Towards a Model of Midwifery Management

Diane Brears

Head of Midwifery, Royal Oldham Hospital

Introduction

Thirty years ago Rosemary Stewart (1963) defined management as 'seeing what needs to be done and then getting others to do it'. Today, we talk of vision and leadership. This paper will explore these concepts in relation to midwifery management and the changing environment in which we work.

'Changing Childbirth' (1993) offers exciting opportunities to develop the maternity services in ways that appeal to mothers and midwives. The objectives set out in this blueprint of the future rely upon the goodwill and enthusiasm of midwives, appropriate investment in the service by Purchasers, but perhaps above all upon dynamic and motivated managers. If the changes demanded by the report are to become reality, the requirement for 'clear thinking, real leadership and commitment to commonly shared values' (p.1995) will be paramount.

During periods of rapid change supervision of midwives is an important statutory function, which protects and maintains professional standards consistent with the Midwives Rules and Code of Practice. But it is midwifery managers who set the organizational goals and who ensure organizational success.

A key objective of midwifery management is to achieve a high quality service, which meets contractual obligations. 'Changing Childbirth' objectives form the core of purchaser specifications for the maternity service. But how individual units meet these objectives depends upon the vision, imagination and innovation of midwifery management. There is no single model which all units could or would wish to adopt. Each unit is unique, they serve different local populations with varying demands and priorities. Midwives operate within very different organizational cultures and face variable constraints to practice and professional development. Effective midwifery managers recognize these constraints and endeavour to overcome them. Like Supervisors of Midwives, managers have a duty to facilitate the acquisition of new skills, not only to meet the requirements of the profession in accordance with the statutory bodies, but to meet the requirements of a dynamic, modern service. It is clear that the roles of midwifery managers and Supervisors of Midwives can and do overlap. Anecdotal evidence suggest that the two roles are not always easily separated and that some midwives - managers, supervisors and clinical practitioners - confuse the two.

Recent changes to the preparation of Supervisors of Midwives and more rigorous selection and assessment criteria are a welcome development. These changes acknowledge the special skills needed by Supervisors of Midwives if they are to support and guide their colleagues. The remainder of this paper describes characteristics of effective management. It will be up to the reader to decide if the roles of managers and supervisors are complimentary or not.

Total quality management

Traditional management styles place emphasis on controlling people. In the modern NHS management styles and methods based on effective leadership and total quality principles are needed.

Features of a 'traditional' management style include:

- Short term outlook
- Lack of clear strategy
- Clamping down on costs whilst tolerating high levels of waste
- A 'take it or leave it' attitude to customers
- Discouraging change
- Fire fighting management

This management style is successful only as long as:

- Employees do as they are told
- Demand exceeds supply
- Customers expectations change only slowly
- The 'world' situation does not change
(Department of Trade and Industry, 1991)

As all midwives know, the environment in which we work is rapidly changing. The expectations and demands of service users are constantly rising, financial systems are fluid and unpredictable and many NHS Trusts are fighting to survive. In this environment, maternity services need effective leadership and a clear quality strategy as outlined below.

Principles of effective Leadership:

- Develop clear beliefs and objectives
- Develop clear and effective strategies
- Identify critical processes
- Review management structure
- Encourage effective employee participation

Principles of a quality strategy:

- Satisfy customer needs
- Get close to customers
- Plan to do all jobs right first time
- Agree expected performance standards
- Implement unit wide quality improvement
- Measure performance
- Measure quality lapses and firefighting
- Demand continuous improvements
- Recognize achievements

(Department of Trade and Industry, 1991)

Effective organizations

Mintzberg (1991) proposed that effective managers build effective organizations by managing the interplay of seven basic forces. The following model demonstrates how the principles outlined above can be incorporated into the structure of an organization.

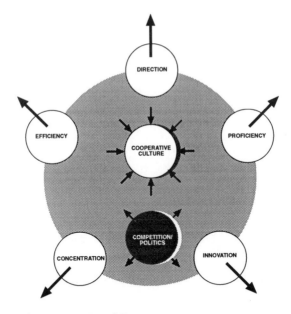

Figure 1. A System of Organizational Force

The first force is *direction* which is the sense of vision and mission for the organization.

The next force is *efficiency* which is the need to minimize costs and increase benefits.

The third force, *proficiency* means carrying out tasks with a high level of knowledge and skill. Maternity Services use highly trained professionals to achieve excellence.

The fourth force is *innovation*, the need to develop new services to adapt to the external environment, i.e. government, purchasers and public opinion.

The fifth force is *concentration* which focuses organizational efforts onto particular 'markets'. In the context of midwifery management the focus has to be upon a woman centred and consumer led maternity service.

Two additional forces within the pentagon of figure 1 are *co-operative culture* and *competition/politics*. Co-operation is the result of common culture values and reflects the need for harmony among health care professionals working within the maternity service. Competition and professional rivalry can damage working relationships and result in the isolation of individuals, departments and/or professional groups.

By understanding these forces and designing the right organizational structure to achieve strategic objectives, midwifery managers can create effective maternity services. This is, of course, a continual leadership process.

Effective leaders

Crainer (1988) described six crucial personality characteristics of effective leaders:

- Need for mastery
- Active, assertive, persistent
- Belief in self
- Goal orientated
- A need for recognition
- Ability to accept need for self development

Huczynski and Buchanan (1991) list the following as desirable qualities of top managers:

- Care   Dependability
- Judgement   Fairness
- Integrity   Foresight
- Energy   Dedication

I believe three factors will come to characterize maternity services:

- Leadership vision
- Bias towards action
- Minimal rationality

Successful maternity services have a special kind of leadership vision which is leadership of the organization, not leadership within it. The leader provides a vision of what can be accomplished and gives a sense of purpose and meaning to staff working within the service. Visionary leaders are involved in key organizational issues and communicate face to face with all employees. They lead by example and push dominant values with a single minded focus.

Successful maternity units are orientated towards doing, towards implementation. A bias towards action means that they don't talk problems to death, they 'do it, fix it, try it'. The management style empowers and supports staff to be innovative and to take calculated risks.

Research into progressive, adaptive organizations indicates they 'minimize rationality' rather than rely on objective, quantitative decision rules (Daft, 1992). In today's rapidly changing environment rational methods may not be fast enough, accurate enough or able to handle ambiguity. Midwifery managers must have the confidence to rely upon their own judgement and instincts.

Conclusion

Midwifery management provides the framework within which clinical practices can be effectively and efficiently carried out. Midwife managers have a primary role to promote and facilitate delivery of care which reflects those values central to individualized care and professionally stated standards.

Quality of service relies essentially on midwives through their individual and collective actions. Midwifery managers need to support and encourage their staff to be innovative, responsive and sensitive to the ever changing needs of the service and those who use it. This can only be achieved through the development of a working environment that values individual contribution and allows midwives to maximise their own potential.

Maternity services of acknowledged excellence depend upon well trained and highly motivated staff. Managers have to believe that staff are their most important resource and that investment in training and continuing education will be reflected in staff morale and quality of care.

The challenges and opportunities presented by 'Changing Childbirth' require midwifery mangers to have vision, leadership skills and a strong and coherent value system. A strong set of beliefs and values shared by managers provides the necessary foundation for coping with uncertainty and managing change. Without effective midwife managers who command the trust and loyalty of their staff 'Changing Childbirth' could be doomed to failure.

This paper has described managerial characteristics and suggested a model for the future. Effective managers support, guide and develop their staff to provide a high quality service. Effective supervisors support, guide and develop individual midwives to promote excellence in practice. They require acknowledged clinical and interpersonal skills. Midwife managers too must have credibility with clinical colleagues and expert interpersonal skills, but in addition they need highly developed business acumen.

My contention is that effective managers can be effective supervisors of midwives, but effective supervisors may not necessarily be effective managers.

References

Cumberledge Report (1993). *Changing Childbirth The Report of the Expert Maternity Group.* London: HMSO.

Crainer, S. (1988). 'Making boss-power positive.' *The Sunday Times.* 9th October .

Daft, R.L. (1992). *Organization Theory and Design* 2nd Ed. New York:West Publishing Co.

Department of Trade and Industry (1991). *Total Quality Management and Effective Leadership.* London.

Huczynski, A. Buchanan, D. (1991). *Organizational Behaviour - An Introductory Test.* 2nd Ed. New York: Prentice Hall.

Mintzberg, H (1991). 'The Effective Organization, Forces and Forms', *Sloan Management Review* Winter 1991 pp.54-67.

Page, L. (1995). *Effective Group Practice in Midwifery, Working with Women,* Oxford: Blackwell Science.

Stewart, R. (1963). *The Reality of Management.* London: Pan Books.

The Consumer View

Beverley Lawrence Beech

Honorary Chairperson AIMS

'The women must be the focus of maternity care. She should be able to feel that she is in control of what is happening to her and able to make decisions about her care, based on her needs, having discussed matters fully with the professionals involved.' (Cumberlege, 1993)

Ask most women during their pregnancy who the Supervisor of Midwives is and she probably will look at you blankly. The majority of women never come across a midwifery supervisor.

Where supervision is good the consumers are completely unaware that it exists. AIMS has supported both women and midwives in cases where the woman has chosen a home birth despite being, justifiably, advised to have her baby in hospital. We have seen how good supervision has given the midwife advice and support and both the woman and the midwives were pleased to have that. We have seen cases where the midwife who feels in need of advice and support will approach her Supervisor, discuss her anxieties, consider the options and the support she needs and, in the majority of cases, the woman has been unaware that this has happened.

Cases of poor supervision claim greater attention and while these cases identify and publicize sub-standard behaviour and are valuable indicators of problems, it is most important that good supervision is identified, and equally publicized, if only to give other supervisors and midwives the opportunity of understanding how good supervision can be encouraged and promoted. Midwives are extremely bad at writing up their good experiences (or, for that matter, the poor ones) and this failure deprives the profession of learning from good examples or addressing the poor ones.

Home birth appears to be the main area where a supervisor of midwives becomes obvious to the woman. While there are many areas of the country where a request for a home birth is treated no differently from a request for a hospital delivery, there are areas where the woman will not only receive a consultation from her midwife but will also be visited in her own home by a supervisor. If every woman had such care we would have to employ thousands of extra supervisors, why is this standard of service not given to women who choose a hospital birth?

AIMS has yet to receive a report of a woman having a hospital delivery being visited at home to have the risks and dangers carefully explained to her, yet for the majority of women the risks of a hospital delivery are greater than those of a home birth (Tew, 1995).

Where care is poor, the woman becomes only too aware of the presence of the Supervisor of Midwives.

Problems with supervision appear, from a consumer viewpoint, to fall into two categories:

1. The mother and the midwife versus the supervisor.

2. The supervisor and the midwife versus the mother.

The first example involves the midwife trying her best to respond to the needs of the woman, and the Supervisor of Midwives acting in an authoritarian, punitive and oppressive manner, so the woman and the midwife end up feeling they are both in a battle of wills. The second example involves a Supervisor and the midwives joining together to 'persuade' the woman to accept their advice and come into hospital.

Mother and midwife versus the supervisor

In April 1993, two midwives, Valerie Foster and Jill Kruzens, booked a woman for a water birth at home. In December 1993, following the publicity about water births from the Royal College of Obstetricians and Gynaecologists, the midwives were informed that they could not offer a water birth as the hospital, Queen Elizabeth II, Welwyn Garden City, did not have a contract to do so.

The Supervisor of Midwives, Freda Kelly, insisted that the midwives instruct the mother to get out of the water for the birth 'as this was Trust policy'. The Supervisor did not appear to be concerned with the fact that the Trust has no jurisdiction whatsoever in a woman's own home and was in no position to dictate anything. Unfortunately, the community midwives omitted to ask the Supervisor what she would advise should the woman refuse to move. They presumed, not unreasonably, that having invited the woman to get out of the water, and having received a refusal, they had a duty to get on with it and deliver the baby. This they did. The following day they found themselves suspended and subsequently disciplined for failing to follow Trust instructions.

The mother, Valerie French, found herself deprived of the care of two midwives who had built up a relationship of trust and rapport and was extremely distressed to find that she was no longer allowed to be attended by those midwives.

It is difficult to understand how care was safeguarded, or even improved, by removing these midwives from duty and depriving a mother of their advice and expertise. As a result of local disciplinary action one of the midwives is still working in hospital, not allowed back onto the district, and the other midwife has sought employment in, one hopes, a more enlightened Health Authority.

Is it right to suspend midwives who are not a danger to the public or whose practise could not be faulted? AIMS has a list of midwives whose practice was highly questionable and, in some cases, positively dangerous, yet no action was taken against them. In some cases, they had a warm and friendly relationship with the supervisor and were rarely known to question anything. Too often we have seen the good, competent, and questioning midwives with high standards being targeted as 'trouble makers' and every effort made to drive them out of the district, if not the profession.

Not only are some Supervisors of Midwives woefully ignorant of parents' rights and the boundaries of their responsibilities, they are also not above lying. An example of this is the Supervisor of Midwives in the Home Counties who would tell her midwives, 'Don't worry about having to do a home birth, just wait until 39 weeks and tell the woman that her blood pressure has increased and she now has to come into hospital, they always do'. Indeed they do, until the grapevine spreads the word and a lone woman makes a fuss and refuses to go in. Unfortunately, in one particular instance, the lone woman really did have an increase in her blood pressure and would have been safer in hospital, but she no longer believed the midwife. That particular midwife was paying the price for her colleagues' previous dishonesty. Fortunately, the outcome was a success, but it did not do the midwife's nor our blood pressure any good at all.

Supervisor and the midwife versus the mother

Childbirth is not a scientific event but a normal life experience. There is, therefore, no way in which care can, or should, be rigidly standardized, and women's experiences over the last 50 years of hospital's attempts to standardize their interventions is testimony to the risks and inappropriateness of much of the care. Every woman has different experiences, different expectations and different problems may emerge during the pregnancy and labour. A good, sensitive, midwife will be aware of the variables and will discuss the options available with the mother, and sometimes approach the Supervisor of Midwives to determine what action could, or should, be taken.

Unfortunately, this approach is not adopted by everyone, and for some women their refusal to accept the advice they have been given is met with hostility and a determination to 'persuade' them to capitulate.

In May, 1992 AIMS was contacted by Jenny Smith, a woman living on the Shetland Islands (Beech, 1994). She wanted a home birth. Such a request in this area, as with most of Scotland, was not met with any support, and as she had had a previous caesarean section the staff felt justified in persisting with their 'advice' that she should give birth in hospital.

They did not hear her reasons why she was not prepared to accept a hospital birth for this baby. She had already experienced the 'benefits' of a hospital delivery, in the Ayrshire Central Hospital, for her first baby; and the experience had traumatized her to the extent that she was determined never to set foot in a hospital again, if she could possibly avoid it.

The story of the previous birth was not anything out of the ordinary, unfortunately.

'From the moment I went to my GP I felt my pregnancy belonged to them. I went to all the antenatal appointments like a good girl. When I went for my first antenatal appointment at the hospital I refused an internal. I wasn't asked but told they were going to do it. Again I refused, but I felt totally humiliated and degraded afterwards. I never had an internal until I was in labour. I refused until then because I saw no point in frequent antenatal internals. From then on I had this deep fear that things were going to go terribly wrong. I was terrified and intimidated every time I went to the hospital. I was scared of the birth and wanted to have the baby at home. I didn't say anything about it as I was sure they would know best. How wrong could I be?'

She went into labour and into hospital. A Registrar decided that the labour was not proceeding fast enough and ruptured the membranes, she had a drip, catheter, and was confined flat on her back, had an epidural, and ended up with six people in the room. The consultant, at 10 centimetres dilation and the baby's head high, declared that she could push for an hour and then it was a forceps or caesarean. She ended up with a caesarean section, a wound infection, and problems bonding with the baby, followed by 14 months postnatal depression. Hardly a surprise that she wanted the next baby at home.

The impact of this birth on her was ignored by the Shetland midwives. Her GP told her that her baby was at high risk and she left his consulting rooms very upset. When she explained her fear of hospitals and what had happened to her he laughed it off and suggested she would know all about postnatal depression if her baby died.

The next day her midwife called, as she had been bleeding, and tried to persuade her how wonderful the local maternity unit was, and suggested that she should see the community psychiatric nurse. This Jenny did and found her to be useless. Sometime afterwards Jenny received a letter from Aileen Anderson, the Supervisor of Midwives, strongly advising a hospital delivery.

The pressure from every professional involved persisted throughout her pregnancy. The staff's attitude was that she was not listening to what they were saying, therefore if they said it often enough, and in a variety of ways, she would soon understand and 'be a good girl'. When she challenged a midwife about the constant pressure the midwife's response was 'well it is for your own good'. Since when is it in any woman's own good to force her into a form of care of which she is afraid? How would these midwives expect her to achieve a normal birth in such circumstances? But they were not expecting her to have a normal birth, they were determined that she was going to have a caesarean section and they were going to do everything possible to ensure that she needed one.

Instead of having a contented and stress free time, she spent most of her pregnancy worrying and anxious about the impending birth. When she went into labour she called the midwives. Liz Cook was the first midwife to arrive. She checked the mother and then called her colleague, Janette Sanderson. The checks continued at intervals, and Jenny was told that she would be given 24 hours after her waters had broken and then she would have to go into hospital. As time progressed the midwives telephoned Aileen Anderson and was told that Aileen had said that she had until 6.00pm and then she would *have* to go into hospital. Unfortunately, Jenny did not realize that the Supervisor of Midwives had no authority to put a time limit on her labour and was exceeding her remit.

The midwives persuaded Jenny to agree to putting the ambulance on standby. As soon as she agreed to this the midwives increased their pressure for her to go into hospital. Shortly afterwards, the front door burst open and two ambulancemen rushed into her home clutching a chair and a stretcher. The midwives carried on about the dangers of continuing to labour at home while a neighbour persuaded the ambulancemen to wait up the road at her home. Jenny dismissed everyone so that she could have some time to speak with her husband. The midwives, in the meantime, packed their equipment and loaded it into the ambulance and their cars. Jenny and her husband decided that they were not going to leave and discovered that the ambulancemen had not been called out on standby – their instructions were to take Jenny into hospital immediately.

When the midwives learned of Jenny's decision not to go into hospital, they were furious and crashed around the house. The GP arrived, he was arrogant and intimidating and wanted to examine her. Jenny refused. The midwife wanted to check her blood pressure and Jenny went with her into the bedroom for this to be done. The GP was asked to leave, which he did after he went into another room to talk to the midwives. Calm descended, the midwives' attitude changed, they became very calm and understanding and Jenny had the feeling that something was afoot.

During this time Gerald, the husband, rang me, in tears. They were having such problems with the midwives and what could they do about it? I advised him to kick the midwives out and insist on getting a more sympathetic midwife. The couple did not feel strong enough to do that. So, I rang the Aileen Allen, the Supervisor of Midwives, to discuss what could be done to try and instil some humanity into the midwives' behaviour and her support of them. She took an hour and a half to return my call. Another AIMS' member, Nadine Edwards, the Secretary of AIMS Edinburgh, also rang, and was met with a self satisfied, hostile, and unfeeling attitude. The Supervisor saw no reason to intervene, the midwives were qualified and dealing with a very difficult case and she certainly was not going to do anything to intervene. I received a similar response when I finally managed to track her down.

It concerned me that having received an urgent call concerning a home birth Aileen Allen did not respond immediately. At the time I contacted her she had no idea who I was and for all she knew I could have been trying to alert her to an imminent disaster. It did not seem to bother her that it took an hour and a half between my urgent phone call and her response.

The AIMS phone calls did nothing to encourage Aileen Allen to consider the effect her staff were having on a labouring woman. In the meantime, having failed to persuade Jenny to go into hospital, the midwives rang the GP, who arrived and tried further persuasion. The couple threw him out.

A short while later he re-appeared, with a consultant psychiatrist. The GP considered that Jenny should be sectioned under the Mental Health Act. To the psychiatrist's considerable credit he discussed the situation with Jenny and pronounced that there was nothing whatsoever the matter with her and he was going home.

With a labour subjected to so much stress it was not surprising that the baby's heart-beat started to fall, and, recognizing that her baby was in need of help, Jenny decided that the time had come for her to go into hospital. The hospital staff treated her very well, particularly the consultant surgeon. She had a caesarean section and delivered a 7lb 14oz boy.

AIMS advised her to report the Supervisor of Midwives and the community midwives to the Scottish National Board and also report the GP to the Family Health Services Committee. She felt most angry about the GP and duly complained. He wrote a letter of apology. She also wrote to Aileen Anderson complaining about the way she was treated and the breaches of confidentiality (practically everyone on the Island knew about her case, and her husband had even been pestered at work by people who felt he should be 'encouraging' his errant wife to go into hospital). She received a two-line letter back saying her points were noted and not even an attempt to apologize for the dreadful way she had been treated. When Jenny met one of the community midwives some weeks later her reaction was 'Well, we told you so'. No doubt they were thoroughly satisfied with the efforts they had made to ensure that their prophesies would come true.

Official information

In November 1992, AIMS conducted a survey of a random selection of English, Welsh and Scottish Health Authorities to try and discover what information they gave their midwives about home birth. We were concerned by the high levels of misinformation which were commonly uttered by midwives and supervisors of midwives. It was not long before we understood why.

It is not unreasonable for midwives to assume that official information they are given is accurate and up-to-date. Unfortunately, our survey revealed otherwise (Beech, 1993).

Altogether AIMS contacted eighteen Health Authorities, Trusts and Health Boards. Six did not reply, despite reminders. The information supplied to midwives varied: eight pages of instructions from the South Devon Health Trust; the Borders Health Board (Scotland) and the Southern Health and Social Services Board (Northern Ireland) provided seven pages of guidance, yet the Northern Health and Social Services Board, and adjacent Health Authority, only one page.

Misunderstandings about the law and home birth are not uncommon. It is not helped when a Health Trust muddies the waters.

'There appears to be a misunderstanding in certain quarters that when a woman becomes pregnant and the time of delivery is near, it is permissible for her and her partner or friend to decide to conduct the birth themselves in their own home without any professional assistance. It should be clearly understood by all concerned that it is an offence for an unqualified person to attend a mother in childbirth except in cases of urgency or emergency. It should also be clearly understood by all concerned that when the parents take deliberate action to conduct the delivery of the baby by themselves in their home this constitutes an offence. The object of the law is to ensure that proper professional treatment is immediately available for the care of the mother and baby on what can be a difficult and dangerous occasion.'

This carefully worded statement which was apparently given to everyone who asked for a home birth, omitted to mention that it is the attendants who commit the illegal act. It is not illegal (although very unwise) for a woman to deliver her baby herself. One wonders why this level of intimidation is necessary, and whether any attempts have been made to establish why some parents reject professional advice? It appears that the Health Trust sees this issue as a failure of parents to take up their services, instead of a failure of the services to respond to the needs of the parents.

It was this same Trust which advised their midwives to 'follow hospital procedures adapting them to home circumstances as necessary.' One presumed that meant, breaking the waters, refusing to allow the woman to eat, watching the clock and requiring the labour to fit into a rigid timetable. Any midwife who seriously followed that advice would be taking considerable risks, and she would not have the friendly obstetric staff down the corridor to rescue her from the potential disaster she has just created.

A supervisor's perspective

In January this year Midwives published an article about a Supervisor's views of the current issues in water birth (Keane, 1995). It is a classic example of how professionals can misunderstand the law, ethics and women's rights and yet be utterly confident of their position. The article highlights Emily's experiences. Emily wants to use water for pain relief and also give birth in it. As no babies had been born in water at Leeds General Infirmary Emily was willing to be used as a 'guinea pig'. If the staff would not 'allow' it she would hire a pool and have the baby at home.

The Supervisor, Heather Keane, felt that Emily's offer to be a guinea pig was unacceptable. She quoted Dimond who points out that,

'if a midwife is not trained in waterbirth delivery and makes an error – which a trained midwife would not have made – then the midwife would be negligent and could not be exempted from liability by pointing out that in her letter Emily had agreed to be a guinea pig. Therefore, not only would the supervisor not be protecting the public (Emily) against poor standards of midwifery practice, she would also be putting midwives at risk of disciplinary action for not abiding by the Midwives Rules... and putting the trust in a position where it could be sued for negligence.'

This line of argument ignores the fact that Keane had time to ensure the midwives were trained, could buy in a trained midwife, and there is a world of difference between 'making an error' and negligence. Furthermore, as Jean Robinson has pointed out in her critique (1995) what action did the midwives in Leeds take when they were faced with the first 'guinea pig' to use ultrasound scan, the first electronic fetal monitoring, the first induction of labour? Were these issues raised then?

Keane goes on to state that,

> 'There is a duty to ensure that Emily's partner did not break the law by contravening the Nurses, Midwives and Health Visitors Act of 1979 (Section 17) by being at the birth and having no qualified midwife or medical practitioner present. There is no duty, the law merely requires a birth to be attended by a qualified medical practitioner or midwife, it makes no demands of the midwifery profession to act to prevent an incident, other than a duty to provide a midwife should one be requested.'

It seems, from Keane's point of view that Emily was between a rock and a hard place. She was not allowed to have a water birth in hospital and a water birth at home was not acceptable as it would be unattended (Keane being unwilling to 'allow' her untrained midwives to attend). Had Emily decided to stay at home one presumes she would have done so believing that she was not entitled to a midwife, as Keane had intimated that she could not allow her untrained midwives to attend and break what she perceived as the rules. Had this scenario occurred, Keane would have found herself in court on a charge of breaking the law as the law clearly requires her to provide a midwife.

It appears that in Leeds the decision to 'allow' a water birth rests with the obstetrician. He has no authority to take this decision and it is puzzling that the midwives have accepted his interference in a matter which does not concern him. Clearly, Keane is unaware of the UKCC Position statement on waterbirth which states,

> 'Waterbirth should, therefore, be viewed as an alternative method of care and management in labour and as one which must, therefore, fall within the duty of care and normal sphere of practice of a midwife. Waterbirth is not considered to be a "treatment".'

Keane offered a solution to her dilemma, she would undertake the delivery (although she does not mention what training she had) and a midwife who had studied water birth would be present too. Should Keane not be available at the time of the birth Emily was asked to agree to leave the pool and give her agreement in writing. If Emily refused to leave the pool, the on-call supervisor was to be informed. What that supervisor was meant to do in those circumstances was not made clear. The problem did not arise, however, as Emily 'decided not to use water as her chosen method of pain relief'. Such a decision makes one wonder just how much pressure was put on Emily to conform to the usual practices in Leeds.

There is an underlying assumption in the article that there is a means of preventing any chance of litigation or disciplinary action by rules and regulations, and signing pieces of paper. Certainly, rules and regulations provide a framework for practice and a yardstick by which one can measure good practice, but it should never be forgotten that litigation can only be taken for acts of negligence (or assault), and no amount of rules and regulation will protect anyone from a person who acts negligently. In circumstances where the midwives have never undertaken a particular procedure before, they have a duty to learn as much about it as they can and act in a professional manner and not in a negligent way (i.e. want of proper care or attention).

Keane's article is a classic example of the way in which the law and midwifery rules can be misinterpreted and misunderstood and used to deny women the right to choose. This article illustrates very well how midwives can fail put the needs of the patient first and by so doing fail to meet the UKCC Code of Practice, which requires a midwife to 'act always in such a manner as to promote and safeguard the interests and well being of patients and clients'.

Midwives' behaviour

It is often quoted that some doctors are drawn to obstetrics because it offers them almost unlimited opportunities to exercise power and control. But the same opportunities are offered to midwives. Why do some midwives behave the way they do, why are some power hungry controllers, why do others in positions of power act like the Midwife from Hell, not only making life a misery for the women in her care but also make life hell on earth for the midwives in her employment? Why are so many midwives silently compliant?

In the AIMS' Journal last year, the editor, Pat Thomas, explored the reasons why midwives are attracted to midwifery and what emotional baggage they bring to their practice and how that affects their care (Thomas, 1994). She produced some startling statistics about women:

- 1 in 3 has been sexually abused
- 3 in 10 is bulimic
- 2 in 10 is or has been anorexic
- 3 in 10 suffers from depression
- 1 in 50 experiences chronic violence in the home
- 1 in 25 is estimated to drink alcohol to an extent which suggests psychological and/or physical dependence
- 1 in 250 women use or have used hard drugs such as cocaine and heroin
- 7.9 in 1000 mothers will experience a stillbirth or the death of a baby in the first week of life
- Nearly 4 in 10 marriages will break up
- It's estimated that some 12 per cent are lesbian or bisexual (though no clear consensus on this has been reached)
- Although there are no accurate figures, a growing number of women are positively choosing to be celibate.

These figures are startling. How could they affect practice? Margaret Logue researched the incidence of post-partum haemorrhage by registrar. She discovered that the rates of this varied by registrar from 1 per cent to 31 per cent. She concluded that,

'Having known and worked with all of these registrars their haemorrhage rates seem to be a reflection of their individual personality: the more conservative and patient operators show the lowest rates compared with the more impatient and heavy-handed who show the highest rates.'

When she repeated the research amongst the midwives, she found a similar range (Logue, 1990).

Why are some midwives impatient? What are the effects on practice of a midwife who was sexually abused as a child, or a midwife who has difficulty dealing with the sexuality of childbirth? Is she more likely to carry out an episiotomy, is she more likely to use drugs? Who knows? It is an issue that has not yet been addressed.

References

Beech, B.A.L. 'We told you so, birth at home and the Mental Health Act' *AIMS Journal*, Vol. 6, No. 3, pp.10–12.

Beech, B.A.L. (1993). 'Guidelines for home birth' *AIMS Journal*, Vol. 5 No. 2, pp. 4–7.

Keane, H. (1995). 'The waterbirth experience, a supervisor's perspective' *Midwives*, January, pp. 9–11.

Logue, M. (1990). 'Management of the third stage of labour. A midwife's view' *Journal of Obstetrics and Gynaecology* 10, Suppl. 2, S10-S12.

Robinson, J. (1995). 'Emily's choice' *AIMS Journal*, Vol. 7 No. 1, pp. 4–5.

Thomas, P. (1994). 'Accountable for what?' *AIMS Journal*, Vol. 6 No.3, pp. 1–5.

Audit of the Supervision of Midwives in the North West Region

Jean Duerden

Introduction

Supervision of Midwives has been operating in various fashions for 93 years and yet research into this area has been very scant and little has been recorded. Jane Tyrer[1], Executive Director/Chief Nursing Adviser for the former Mersey Regional Health Authority, was far sighted enough early in 1994 to set up an audit of the supervision of midwives. As the two regions (Mersey and North Western) were to amalgamate in April she felt it appropriate to carry out this audit across the new North West Region and sought a project leader to undertake this task. I was privileged to be released from my position of midwifery manager and supervisor of midwives for Salford Royal Hospitals NHS Trust for one year from October 1994 to carry out the audit. Mrs Tyrer was keen to ensure that the wider context of supervision of practice for all professionals should also be taken into consideration as preceptorship is introduced and supervision of clinical practice is closely looked at by the nursing profession.

Summary

An audit of supervision of midwives is currently being conducted throughout the North West Region. This one year project is due for completion at the end of September, 1995. Midwives, supervisor of midwives and midwife teachers are interviewed by the project leader in every maternity unit and college of midwifery throughout this large Region, using a structured questionnaire. The results of the audit will be presented at a conference in June and a report will be published in September.

To date sixteen maternity units and four midwifery education establishments have been audited. These visits started with the link supervisors' units so that they could evaluate reception of the audit and ensure that it was unobtrusive, and acceptable to midwives and supervisors alike.

Origin of the project

Central to the NHS reforms is the delivery of a quality health service, which gives choice to users, enables purchasers and providers of care to be responsive to user's needs and ensure a better service. Audit of clinical care is a method of professional self-improvement, but at its root lies the aim of advance of quality of care delivered to patients and clients. This is the philosophy of clinical audit which is suited to an audit of supervision of midwives.

The 1989 White paper 'Working for Patients' led to the establishment of a number of programmes covering medical audit. In June 1991 the Department of Health initiated a three year audit programme for nursing and therapy professions. Clinical audit money was distributed to each Regional Health Authority by the Department of Health, and Regional Clinical Audit Coordinators were appointed.

The programme's aim was to enable clinical audit to become part of a wider quality improvement strategy and was expected to encompass five elements; defining standards of care, defining data requirements and systems, identifying staff concerned with specific audit goals, setting up arrangements to include clinical audit in the overall management process and reviewing procedures.

The goals to be achieved were:

Outcome of audit: improvement in the quality of care and best achievable outcomes.

Infrastructure: clinical audit should be fully embedded in the NHS.

Education and training: audit should be an integral part of all professional education.

National projects: where results should have a wide application and are transferable.

Standards: audit should include standard setting which can be measured against practice.

Purchasing: audit findings should inform the contracting process.

Founding for projects has ranged from a little as a few hundred pounds up to £40,000 for projects running over several years. A total of £17.7 million has been allocated over three years to support nursing and therapy audit. The North West Regional Health Authority has invested £30,000 in the audit of the supervision of midwives.

The audit programmes have been lead in each Region by a clinical Audit Co-ordinator. Their role has been to set up arrangements for funding and monitoring the projects, and to initiate region-wide projects. Audit is being used to bring about change. Specific changes resulting from audit have predominantly concerned improvements to patient care.

Clinical audit has occasionally had poor publicity in some areas but the North West Region is taking the audit of the supervision of midwives very seriously. There is no suggestion that it will be taken as merely a paper exercise.

The terms of Reference are as follows:

1. To undertake a systematic and independent examination of supervision of mid-wives in the new North West Region.

2. To determine whether supervisory activities and related outcomes comply with current guidelines.

3. To determine whether the arrangements for and practice of midwives is consistent and represents value of money.

4. To review and if necessary revise the current guidelines.

5. To produce a final report no later than one year from the commencement of the project.

CASPE Research has been commissioned by the Department of Health to undertake an evaluation of the nursing and therapy audit programmes in the hospital and Community Health Services in England. The audit of supervision of midwives has been included in this survey.

The project method

For the audit tool three interview questionnaires have been devised: a collective interview for all the supervisors about policies and procedures for supervision within the maternity unit, an individual interview for each supervisor of midwives and a similar interview for midwives. The questionnaires were first scrutinized by the Regional Nurse Education and Professional Development and than by all members of the steering group. All suggested amendments which were introduced in the sub-drafts. Nineteen drafts in all were written and piloted. I received excellent support and help from Jane Winship and Jill Steene at the United Kingdom Central Council (UKCC) and Glynnis Mayes at the English National Board (ENB) in the final stages of preparing the questionnaires. The interviews have been structured to ensure that no question is open to misinterpretation and effort has been made to remove the variables. In order to remain objective, the same questions are asked in the same manner.

The first audit took place on October 25th, 1994. There are thirty three maternity units in the North West Region and each unit is included in the audit. As many supervisors of midwives and midwives are interviewed as can be arranged in a one day visit. Each interview takes approximately 15 to 25 minutes with each supervisor of midwives and roughly 15 minutes with each midwife. All the colleges of midwifery in the Region are included in the audit to interview midwife teachers. With co-operation from the heads of midwifery the audit visits should all be completed by the end of April and the evaluation of all the results can commence.

The North West Region covers a large area, being 110 miles north to south and 60 miles east to west on the mainland. This is from as far north as the Lake District, and south as far as Crewe: the distance over the sea, west to the Isle of Man, is in addition to the above measurement. The latter was a particularly interesting visit. Although controlled by their own Department of Health, Manx nursing and midwifery staff are governed by UKCC regulations. Statutory supervision of midwives is therefore the responsibility of the Local Supervising Authority (LSA) at the North West Regional Health Authority.

The information that I am collecting in the audit of the supervision of midwives is a combination of statistical evidence and the opinions of midwives across the region. I am recording all the comments that I receive from both midwives and supervisors of midwives. Already this makes interesting reading. I am also collating 'Good Practice' ideas from each unit which will be valuable to all supervisors of midwives.

The list that follows describes the information received from the interviews:

- Numbers of supervisors of midwives in each unit.
- Number of midwives per supervisor of midwives.
- Supervision records in each unit.
- Supervision arrangements for allocation (managed/not managed).
- Who supervises the supervisors of midwives?
- Who supervisies the Head of Midwifery?
- Arrangements for notification of intention to practise forms.
- Organization of professional updating.
- Responsibility of preceptorship.
- Arrangements for 24 hour access to supervisors of midwives.
- Number of practice nurses practising as midwives.
- Arrangements for supervision of practice nurses practising as midwives.
- Number of independent midwives residing/practicing in the area.
- Arrangements for independent midwives.
- Wider role of supervision of midwives within each unit.
- Grades of supervisors of midwives.
- Roles of supervisors of midwives.
- Methods of supervision of midwifery.
- Frequency of supervisory reviews.
- Time spent on direct supervision of midwives.
- Access to link supervisors of midwives and LSA Officer.
- Contact with supervisors of midwives of other areas.
- Advice and support for supervisory function.
- Preparation of supervisors of midwives.
- Selection for appointment of supervisors of midwives.
- Updating of midwives in neonatal units, colleges, GP practices and management.
- Contact of midwives with the supervisors of midwives.
- Midwives' impressions of supervision of midwives.
- How midwives see their own supervisor of midwives.
- Areas of support required by midwives from their supervisor of midwives.
- Quality of supervision of midwifery given to midwives.
- Midwives and supervisors of midwives choice for method of selection of supervisors.
- Qualities valued in supervisors of midwives.

Outcomes to date

The warmth of welcome that I have received everywhere has been generous and hospitable. On rare occasions there has been slight hostility or suspicion from midwives, but it generally proved that they had an axe to grind. As an auditor I have found myself being used as an 'agony aunt' by all grades of staff. The outsider seems to be a sounding board for many anxious midwives and midwife managers.

To date I have interviewed 172 midwives, 44 midwife teachers and 68 supervisors of midwives. I have interviewed as few as six and as many as eighteen midwives in one session and anything from one to seven supervisors. There are 17 more maternity units to audit and one college of midwifery. I therefore estimate that the final number of midwives interviewed will be in the region of 360, 55 midwife teachers and 140 supervisors of midwives. There are 147 supervisors of midwives in the region and approximately 2,950 midwives and midwife teachers. The audit will therefore have involved approximately 95 per cent of supervisors of midwives and midwife teachers. The results of the audit will be ready for presentation at the audit of Supervision of Midwives Conference, an ENB approved study day, on June 22nd, 1995 at the Swallow Trafalgar Hotel in Samlesbury, Preston and in written report form in September, 1995. Both the UKCC and the ENB will be represented in at the conference, Glynnis Mayes, Assistant Director, Midwifery Supervision the ENB and Sarah Roch, Chairman of the UKCC Midwifery Committee, are the keynote speakers.

From the audits I have already completed I am in the process of producing statistical evidence about how midwives and supervisors of midwives feel about the selection of supervisors and the qualities required. The evidence will be reported to the North West Region's working group on selection of supervisors of midwives.

Anticipated outcomes

The anticipated outcomes of the audit are to be able to demonstrate that supervisory activities and related outcomes comply with current guidelines and the arrangements for and practice of supervision is consistent and represents value for money. Outcome measures are that the audit should be able to inform the profession of the reliability and validity of supervision with equal access to supervision and to demonstrate the effectiveness of link supervision. Finally, supervision is credible for all nursing staff and a target for the future – but should the midwifery model be used?

Conclusion

The general impression, so far, is that supervision is alive and well in the North West Region. A midwife is yet to be interviewed who is unaware of supervision or her supervisor. Very few midwives believe that they do not need supervision. Fewer than expected view supervision negatively.

Footnotes

1. Jane Tyrer is the former Regional Nurse Adviser, North West Region

2. Jean Faugier was appointed Regional Nurse Adviser, North West Region from October, 1994

Acknowledgements

Salford Royal Hospitals NHS Trust
North West Regional Health Authority

References

Department of Health (1994). *Clinical Audit in the Nursing and Therapy Professions*. London.
UKCC (1990). *The Report of the Post Registration Education and Practice Project*. London: UKCC.
UKCC (1993). *The Council's Position Concerning a Period of Support and Preceptorship*. (Registrar's Letter 1/1993.) London: UKCC.
Butterworth, C.A., Faugier[2] J. (1992). *Clinical Supervision and Mentorship in Nursing*, London: Chapman and Hall.

Psychodynamic Counselling and Therapy

Meg Taylor

BSc, Msc, RM, Dip Couns

In this paper I have decided to operate almost entirely from my own experience as a counsellor and supervisee rather than to refer to other authorities. As a trainee in both counselling and psychotherapy, I have had three years experience of group supervision, one year of individual supervision and some sessions of peer supervision. As a practitioner, I have had six years experience of individual supervision. I have had three different group supervisors, from different theoretical backgrounds and two individual supervisors, both from a psychoanalytic background. I have also spent many years as a client in therapy. What follows is therefore personal and I take full responsibility for any quirks in my interpretation of theoretical concepts.

Before considering supervision it seems necessary to decide what counselling is and to explain why there may be confusion in the text between counselling and psychotherapy. The distinction between the two is very hard to define. One psychotherapist I met said that if a client goes to a counsellor she cannot necessarily assume that the counsellor has had experience of counselling, whereas all psychotherapists should have had experience of therapy. I practise both and my working distinction is that counselling is what I do with a client who comes with a clearly defined problem and with whom I work for a limited number of sessions decided in advance; psychotherapy is longer, open ended and allows more opportunity to build up a deeper relationship with the client. Occasionally I will use the words therapy and therapeutic, particularly because the psychodynamic theory I use in both counselling and therapy is more common in therapy than counselling. This theoretical approach is not the only one. Another writer coming from a different perspective would produce a very different paper. It is possible that within counselling as opposed to psychotherapy that my approach is a minority one.

In its Resources Directory for 1991 the British Association for Counselling described counselling as: 'a process which involves the helping skills of caring, listening and reflecting. It's based on listening to the client and a trusting relationship between the client and the counsellor. It's not the same as advice giving. A counsellor will be supportive, but will give little or no direct advice, since the aim of counselling is to help us develop our own insight into our problems.' I find this a bland description which doesn't seem to touch on the skills necessary to practise counselling. I want to be clear about the difference between using counselling skills and counselling. Counselling skills include 'caring, listening and reflecting' and an experienced midwife conducting a booking interview, for example, will use them. But she will not be counselling the woman. In addition to the development of the special relationship between counsellor and client, which I will describe in detail below, counselling is marked by a clear bounded structure to the sessions and by a contract between counsellor and client. A woman being booked by a midwife using counselling skills will experience 'being booked' and should feel attended to and heard, but she should not, however complex and difficult her circumstances, become embroiled in more: she has not consented to it. A client in counselling, however has clearly contracted to a part of the counselling process.

Counselling and therapy are very odd. Two people sit together in a room and engage in something quite different from a conversation. The client does most of the talking, the counsellor says very little and may not even respond. There may be long periods of silence. Normal rules of politeness are irrelevant and, understandably, emotions in the client, especially anxiety, run high. The counsellor is also experiencing often intense emotion, however imperturbable she may seem. Areas of life which are usually taboo are brought to light. Searingly painful past experiences may be confronted and expressed. It is not an easy thing to engage in and anyone may reasonably ask why we do it. The answer for me is that on a basic level the use of counselling skills can help the client to solve problems and on a deeper level the development of the therapeutic relationship can bring about profound change.

While counsellors do use and build on the basic counselling skills of caring, listening and reflecting, they do so within this distant framework of bounded sessions, with the client's clear consent to the process. Setting this up; the ability to tolerate and accept silence, uncertainty, negative feelings and pain, the development of the unique relationship of counsellor and client – these seem to me the skills necessary to practise counselling which the BAC description omits.

I consider the peculiar relationship between counsellor and client to be of prime importance both in work with the client and in supervision. I want to look at the two fairly technical aspects of transference and counter transference because the latter is what, in my opinion, supervision is all about and I can't explain counter transference without first looking at transference.

The counselling relationship is not like friendship or love, it is professional. It only happens in reality at certain defined times, although the relationship continues in the minds of both client and counsellor outside those times. Almost always the client pays for it. It is very one sided – the client is vulnerable and while there is debate on how much a counsellor may legitimately reveal of herself, the client will always be hugely more exposed. Clients do not see their counsellor as she really is, they experience *transference*. This is sometimes caricatured as falling in love with the therapist. It may involve this, but it will certainly involve the client's revealing and re-enacting whatever is her most deeply embedded mode of relating to others. This re-enacting is so powerful it will override factors of race or gender for example. With my last therapist, an Indian man, I found myself compulsively reacting as though he was my white Anglo-Saxon Protestant mother. My experience is that we each have a core dynamic, a template for how we make relationships. This template is forged very early on. As midwives we know that all the skills and preferences babies are born with – the grasp and sucking reflexes, the fixed focus of about nine inches that brings the mother's face into clear sight when the baby is at the breast, the preference for looking at faces over anything else – are social and are the basis for relationship making. The quality of the mother's response shapes the template which develops further as the child gets older within the broader relationships of the family and society. I am open to the idea that antenatal events can be influential to a greater or lesser degree. One antenatal event of undeniable importance is conception when each individual's unique genetic endowment is created. Different significant others will evoke different patterns, but these early patterns will be deeply embedded and difficult to change.

Transference is always revealed in counselling (and in other relationships, especially when dependency is an issue: midwives receive a lot of transference from their clients). This revelation to begin with is unconscious. The client does not intend to perceive and relate to the counsellor as she has done to significant others in the past, nor does she know she is doing it. The extent to which I refer to or work on the transference depends on what the client wants from me. If a client wants five sessions to explore why she feels so stuck at work and whether she should make a career move then I would not focus on the transference, although I might refer to it. If a client has come for therapy to work through a past experience of sexual abuse, for example, then after sufficient time has elapsed to build up a relationship of trust between us the work would become 'with the transference' – in other words I would use the experience we undergo in the session to make immediate and real the client's habitual patterns of response. This way of working brings the past into the here and now. There are many explanations as to how this is therapeutic. The one that makes most sense to me from my experience as a client in therapy is that it brings me face to face with long buried pain which I can then express and survive. I found myself in therapy sobbing with grief for my father who had died thirty years previously. This outpouring had a quality of real physical release; in fact the word catharsis means purging in Greek. But it wasn't just the release of such long held tension that was healing but the sense that I had overcome and survived whatever it was that had prevented me from expressing the grief all those years ago. It also offers me the opportunity to become aware of unhelpful habitual responses, such as surpressing my feelings, and to change them. This is hard to do just on the basis of a conscious act of will. What helps is the chance to respond differently in the present therapeutic relationship and to derive a different way of living through pain. Indeed the therapist does not let the client get away with falling back on the old habitual responses.

This transference is not inferred from the overt spoken material of the client alone. It is partly based on this and partly on non-verbal cues and partly on the counsellor's own 'feeling sense' of the session. This feeling sense is *counter transference*. There is debate in psychoanalytic circles about whether this term should be used in the way

I am going to use it or whether it should be restricted to a more technical sense to mean only those responses evoked in the counsellor which get in the way of her being able to help her client. I am going to use it more broadly to mean anything that the clients stirs up in the counsellor. This stirring up is very complex and will include:

1. the therapist's personal habitual ways of responding, which may or may not be helpful and which may or may not be conscious;

2. the client's unconscious ability to cause the therapist to feel what she herself is feeling but is unaware of and cannot therefore express verbally (projective identification);

3   the client's unconscious ability to cause the therapist to feel what other significant people in her life have felt towards her.

I must reiterate that all this is based very much on feeling and intuition and it is an important part of the process to test out intuitions both with clients and in supervision. In case these examples seem too abstract, I shall consider two examples.

One example of how my stuff can intrude in my relationship with a client involves the dynamics of envy and competition. It has become apparent to me during training and therapy that I am a very envious and competitive person. This became troublesome with one particular client. Her success as a nurse contrasted with what might be seen as my failure as a no longer practising midwife. In addition she also was highly competitive and this triggered my own envy and desire to compete. At times I found myself almost sabotaging the therapy so that she did not forge ahead. This unhelpful dynamic was the focus of much supervision.

A clear example of projective identification occurred when I was inexperienced. I had internalized an impossible ideal that I should be warm and compassionate at all times. In a first session with one client I felt intensely, physically frozen and paralysed. The client seemed very much at ease, she was an experienced client and had worked for some time with a previous counsellor. I was confused and felt guilty and inadequate. Rather sheepishly I described this to my supervisor who, I think, I expected to share my sense that I had been insufficiently warm. Instead she seemed almost pleased and explained that all the reactions I felt in a session said something about what was going on with the client and that maybe the frozen paralysis was a reflection of my client's unconscious state of fear. I found this idea that what ever I experienced was valid to be immensely liberating and it formed the basis for my understanding of counter transference.

On both occasions I used supervision to illuminate what was going on. What then is supervision in counselling and psychotherapy, and what does it do?

Just as in midwifery, there are objections to the word 'supervision'. Some prefer to call it 'consultancy'. I don't like the term, it feels too business like and also I believe it is an attempt to deny what for me is a valuable aspect of supervision, namely that my supervisor and I are not equals: she has more experience and a sounder theoretical base that I do. Otherwise I would not be in supervision with her. I quite like the term supervision which comes from the Latin 'to look over' and suggests to me not that my supervisor is looking over my shoulder but that we are both looking over my work. The BAC requires its practising members to be in continual supervision. This, I believe, is unusual. In other countries and in psychoanalytic circles in this country, supervision seems to be reserved for students. Essentially a student or practitioner makes a contracted relationship with a more experienced person or a peer for regular sessions in which aspects of her work will be discussed. Supervision may be individual or group. The frequency will depend on the workload and may be as often as weekly. The theoretical base of the supervision will strongly influence the style of the supervision. It is possible to make a case for choosing a supervision from a different theoretical background. I had this experience as a student and it helped me to clarify my own theoretical beliefs. As a practitioner now, though, it is important that my supervisor shares the same theoretical language as me.

The relationship between supervisor and supervisee mirrors that of counsellor and client to some extent. Just as the counsellor endeavours to create a space where the client can feel safe enough to let her vulnerabilities surface, so that the supervisor creates a degree of trust such that the supervisee can reveal her anxieties, problems, mistakes. The word 'non-judgmental' is often used in counselling. It is a word I dislike because I believe it sets up the kind of impossible ideal of perfection that plagued me when I was a beginner. We all make judgements all the time. I prefer the word 'non-condemnatory' and this expresses the attitude which I have experienced in good supervision.

Supervisory relationships just like any other are not perfect and supervision has its pitfalls. Many beginners are intimidated and afraid to reveal shortcomings for fear of condemnation. It took me a while to realize that supervision involves an almost enthusiastic attitude to error. My supervisor's response to my disclosure about feeling frozen paralysis was not condemnation but a real interest and an expectation that we would examine this as a fascinating manifestation of the process and not as a fault in me. On the other hand, supervisory relationships can get too cosy and insufficiently challenging. I found this a problem in an all-female peer supervision group where it seemed we were all competing to be supportive and on the way lost the opportunity for constructive criticism. The danger of complacency is less in group supervision: more people make collusion less likely. But one problem with group supervision is that the dynamic of the group can become too strong and overwhelm the task of the supervision. Peer groups avoid the problem of intimidation but they miss out on the opportunity of learning from a more experienced person. They are also possibly more vulnerable to being overwhelmed by the group dynamics since they lack a facilitator to clarify what is going on. In any case, groups offer less concentrated time than individual sessions.

Hawkins and Shohet describe six modes of supervision divided into two sub-groups:

A: the therapy session is reported and reflected upon.
    1: focuses on the content of the client's material.
    2: focuses on the responses of the counsellor.

3: focuses on the process of counselling and the relationship between counsellor and client.

B: the therapy process is examined as it is reflected in supervision.
4: focuses on the therapists countertransference.
5: focuses on the here and now of supervision as a possible parallel or mirror of what goes on between counsellor and client.
6: focuses on the supervisor's countertransference.

In my experience a typical supervision session will start by my introducing some aspects of 1, 2 and/or 3 and we will use 4, 5 and/or 6 to clarify whatever the issue might be. We slip in and out of all of these modes in any one session. But for me focusing on countertransference is the most important because it is counter transference that I use almost like an instrument in sessions with a client. For me a major aim of supervision is to enable me to keep my feeling responses to the client as uncontaminated by my personal processes as possible.

One example of a small part of a supervision session went as follows. I was reporting what my client had said (mode 1) and how I had responded (mode 2). After a while my supervisor asked me to reflect on what was going on between us (mode 5). I realized that I had been talking in a flat monotone, staring out of the window and making no attempt to engage her in what I was saying. I felt both bored and boring. So we then looked at what my behaviour said about what was going on with my client (mode 5). Did I find her boring? (mode 4). I didn't think so; rather I thought that by looking out of the window and droning on I was obliquely expressing an angry desire to shut my supervisor out and this reflected what I felt my client did to me (mode 3 and mode 4). Entirely unconsciously I had recreated one aspect of the therapy session in the supervision session. It was my supervisor's countertransference which led her to interrupt me (mode 6). We then went on to question what might lie behind this angry exclusion and how it might be dealt with in future sessions (mode 2 and 3).

In addition to working on Hawkins and Shohet's six levels I find supervision valuable because it offsets the loneliness of the work. I work alone, at home and the contents of all sessions are confidential except to my supervisor. I cannot emerge from a session to confide my responses to what may have been the painful sharing of horrendous abuse. I cannot moan and gossip about a difficult client. Instead I store it up for supervision, although by the time supervision comes along it has usually lost its intensity.

Supervision also helps me to 'contain' the pain. If I am really to listen I cannot metaphorically shut my ears to anything my client may say. Containing here does not mean shutting it up in a box but being able to tolerate what is intolerable to my client until such time as she can take it on board herself. Clients may be able to talk about something but not yet ready to feel it. In theory, and in practice, my training, own experience of therapy and the ongoing support of supervision as well as the tight boundaries of time and space which demarcate the session from the rest of my life enable me to respond compassionately much of the time. The analogy is with the mother of a newborn. The baby who is too young to have a sense of time, place or person knows only that he is starving right now and is crying in panic. His mother, who is confident of her ability to soothe him does not meet panic with panic but calmly (even though no mother can hear her baby cry with equanimity) proceeds to feed him. If the mother is stressed, however, or unsupported then her capacity to meet her baby's needs will be reduced. Supervision provides one of the supports that enables me to avoid meeting panic with panic.

I do not know how relevant this is for midwives. I recently heard Caroline Flint speak at a meeting on supervision. In her opinion midwives, if they are to have clinical autonomy, do not need supervision. I have some sympathy with this point of view and certainly the present set up does seem infantilizing. As far as my practice as a counsellor goes I feel that I have the equivalent of clinical autonomy and that supervision provided the main forum for me to develop it. But the ethos of counselling is very different from that of midwifery and so is the context: I do not practise counselling under the shadow of a more powerful profession whose values are very different from my own. Counselling is considerably less hierarchical and more supportive than midwifery, and while dynamics of competition and envy exist in counselling as everywhere else they are more openly acknowledged and therefore less damaging. One possible danger I see is that midwives may set up supervisory structures which recreate the authoritarianism present in the existing hierarchies. Just as counselling supervision mirrors counselling, so midwifery supervision will mirror midwifery. If a midwifery supervisor can facilitate openness and trust, her supervisee will have more confidence in her own judgements and be able to be open and trusting with the women she supports and towards the process of birth. But if there are condemnatory attitudes and rigid hierarchies supervision will come to feel persecutory and midwives will be unforthcoming.

Any supervision midwives will develop must reflect their own priorities, but I should like to make a plea for midwives to develop their understanding of psychodynamics. I do not mean to imply that any supervisory structures midwives may set up must deal only or primarily with the psychodynamics of their practice but I believe that everything has a psychodynamic (and social) aspect, even for example an emergency caesarean section. Obviously at a time of emergency it is inappropriate to focus on anything other than the task at hand but it may well be relevant and instructive to examine these aspects in supervision. I have always found strong parallels between midwifery and psychotherapy. I am very grateful that I can bring my experience as a midwife, both its practice and philosophy, to my therapeutic work. Midwives 'contain' the pain of women in labour. Just as a midwife does not take the pain of labour away but helps the woman to confront, transform and survive it, because it is the source of the pain that does the work, so a therapist does not deflect a client from pain. If I can 'contain' pain therapeutically, it is largely because I learnt how to be with women in labour. But we all know that midwives differ in their ability to tolerate a labouring woman's pain and some may encourage analgesia to suppress their own empathetic response. As a researcher into emotional aspects of childbearing and their impact on midwifery practice, I believe that midwives might benefit from greater awareness of the unconscious processes influencing their work. This would be asking midwives to look at things from a new angle. But just as I found it liberating to realize that my responses in a session could not be wrong since they would always throw light on the process, midwives might be relieved to interpret the real regression and dependency some women experience as transference, or to perceive some aspects of antenatal care or the use of unnecessary interventions and technology in labour as devices to alleviate professionals' anxiety by minimizing uncertainty and giving an illusion of control.

If midwives are to implement 'Changing Childbirth' they will need to reorientate somewhat, since the language and concepts of changing childbirth are not biomedical but psychological. In any case good supervisory support whatever its focus will produce more confident, assertive midwives and enhance clinical autonomy. The question, it seems to me, is: do midwives need a system of *formal* support structures?

References
British Association for Counselling Resources Directory 1991. British Association for Counselling, 1 Regent Place, Rugby CV21 2PJ.

Hawkins, P., Shohet, R. (1989). *Supervision in the HelpingProfessions*. Buckingham: Open University Press.

Supervision in Social Work

Geoffrey Seaman
BA (Hons), CQSW

Introduction
The available research material
There are available to the serious student or avid reader of social work, many articles, books, research papers and the like, sufficient to satisfy the most dedicated of academics and inform the recently qualified social worker freshly out of college and successfully in her first social work job, just what she might expect from Supervision.

In this paper I will not attempt to summarize this wealth of information, instead I can refer you to a book *Performance Review and Quality in Social Care.* In this collection of research articles there is a chapter by Malcolm Payne entitled 'Personal Supervision in Social Work' which lists 35 references and has a bibliography of 31 articles and books some of which I have read and some not. There is something for every taste and I leave it entirely up to you as to the choice of material to peruse.

The author's background
I must confess from the outset that I am not an academic, although I did obtain an Honours Degree in Applied Social Studies in addition to my Diploma in Social Work some 17 years ago.

I was a social worker in Rotherham and Sheffield from 1978 to 1987, before becoming a Team Leader/Manager in Northumberland until 1991.

Then I took up my present post as a Duty Manager on the Lothian Regional Council Emergency Duty Team which operates outwith normal office hours providing a social work service to 750,000 people in Edinburgh and the Lothians.

What this means is that I have received supervision as a student social worker and then as a qualified practitioner.

I have given supervision as a social worker to students on placement.

I have received supervision from my Area Officer when I was a team leader in which role I had supervisory responsibility for up to 12 staff.

In my present role I meet monthly to discuss my work with my manager whilst myself supervising seven staff on a regular, monthly basis. In addition I have total supervisory responsibility for those shifts that I manage and this means supervising staff as they are in the process of providing an emergency social work service.

It sounds quite tiring just reading about it so how and what do we social workers do in supervision?

The truth is that supervision is varied in terms of frequency, quality, purpose and many other variables. In different social work settings it will be done within groups or teams as opposed to the classic one to one. Staff who work in a residential or day care setting with a particular client group will have different needs and expectations from a social worker in a local office who deals with many client groups and a myriad of problems. This paper will concentrate on illustrating aspects from my own experience as a field worker and team manager, the vast bulk of which has been individual supervision.

Supervision; Many parts make the whole

Most writers comment that supervision has two purposes; firstly a *management* function, secondly a *professional* function which will include an educational or developmental element in it directed at the worker receiving the supervision.

It sounds very simple does it not? Such distinctions are all very well if you are sitting in one of our many fine educational establishments and the simplicity of them can assist in evaluating what social workers and their managers make of and say about the supervisory process. My experience is that the process of supervision is not so easily compartmentalized. I shall return to this theme throughout this paper.

Let us briefly look at the division between managerial and professional in the context of academic research about social work supervision before moving out into the real world and what actually goes on.

(1) *Managerial aspects* will include the social worker's *accountability for their work* - have they actually done the visits they were allocated? Is the social worker being efficient in their use of time? Are assessments accurate and do they indicate what should follow on from the initial contacts between worker and client? Is the worker acting in the best interests of her employing agency in her casework? Is she *following set procedures* as laid down in the Matrix (manuals) which provide guidance and also instruction for staff?

Managerial concerns will look at the volume of work done and whether the worker is doing sufficient. Case load measurement systems were all the rage in the 1970s and 1980s when managers sought to quantify the volume of work being done and compare one worker to their team colleagues or other departmental employees.

You will no doubt recall the DHSS Enquiries into cases of Child deaths (Maria Colwell, Jasmine Beckford etc.) in the 1970s and 80s and that the excuse of overwork was mentioned. Social work was not practised in the art of measurement at that time and substantiating claims of being too busy and having too much too cope with was unconvincing.

Yet it is possible to run a caseload measurement system within a team and I did so in my first management job. I was grateful to my mentor in Northumberland, Alex McGregor, for stressing to me when I arrived, the importance of prioritising the supervision of staff and pointing me to an article by Ann Vickery (1977) on caseload measurement, which sufficed for me.

Recently there has been a new word on the block - *appraisal* or in its newest form *performance review*. This too would come under the heading of a managerial function as it relates to the worker's ability to adhere to the agency procedures and policies i.e. are they doing what they are told to do and then, are they doing it well?

Appraisal also assesses whether or not they are giving value for money and a quality service to clients (service users? – customers!).

The process of appraisal can cross over into the professional area as it may well be part of an assessment of the worker's ability which leads to constructive plans for training designed to expand areas of competency.

(2) *Professional aspects* cover *giving support to the worker* and *guidance* in an educative way which is designed to help the worker develop.

This is the role that much of the research suggests is preferred by the social worker and the supervisor/manager. Both feel more comfortable with supervision being a helping process designed to promote an improvement in the practice of the social worker.

The supervisor's input will vary according to the experience of the social worker. However it is an error to assume that just because a social worker is well versed in the job and has many years of experience that supervision is unnecessary. A recent article in Community Care quoted a practitioner's view;

> 'I want to be challenged...Because I've been around social work a long time, I think people make assumptions that I know more than I do.' (Kearney, 1994)

There has been a recent tendency to refer to 'consultation' rather than supervision as encapsulating the content of the discussion between manager and social worker who is long in the tooth.

In my own experience the difference is semantics; When the faecal matter hits the fan the social worker wants to be able to say they discussed it in supervision with their manager and any decisions were made jointly!

Going off at a tangent for a minute we can note that there has been a movement towards crucial decisions being made by Case conferences with multi-disciplinary personnel involved, particularly in cases of Child Protection. No doubt some of you as midwives will have attended these and shared in the feelings of guilt and anxiety that can be generated when deciding to remove a child from parents or return a child to a situation containing a high degree of risk.

Here we see that a concern for increasing professionalism in decision making has led social work agencies to extend the sphere of influence when considering crucial decisions in high risk cases. Professional considerations applied to the supervision of such cases have been found wanting and mistakes made.

The result is that the emphasis on the professional aspects and supporting the social worker are made subordinate to the need to manage the work done and ensure that it complies with decisions made at case conferences with the worker following pro-cedures.

Returning to our consideration of professional aspects. The purpose of a regular supervision session will include the development of the social worker. The supervisor will want to assess the ability of staff to carry out complex and demanding pieces of work. This will include a consideration of the social worker's emotional, intellectual and practical ability in the work setting. In analysing the social worker's actions in each case the supervisor will explore not just what the worker has done but also how they felt about their actions, the consequences, problems that follow on etc. The supervisor and social worker can share their thoughts about the quality of the work and how it can be maintained and improved.

The supervisor will be gauging the worker's success in forming therapeutic relationships with clients and her effectiveness in engaging in meaningful interaction, setting goals, working towards them and then reviewing achievements prior to disengagement.

At the same time the supervisor will be managing the social worker to assess those things mentioned in the section covering managerial issues.

The *key to the success of this process* is the same as the key to achieving anything in social work. What it is? You have three guesses;

1. The Time Of Day
2. The Time Of The Month
3. The Relationship

The answer of course is *the relationship*.

Relationships within supervision and how to get them right

Supervision demands a relationship between the participants that facilitates success-ful interaction and outcomes of value.

This does not mean that the social worker and supervisor have necessarily to like each other (although it helps). They do have to acknowledge the realities of their relationship and be committed to achieving results within it. This requires that both parties enter into the supervisory relationship with positive intent.

So what must we do?

Initially there must be agreement about the *purpose* of supervision.

Having got this the parties must then *programme* their meetings. It is my view that supervision is best done on a regular basis so that it needs to be programmed into the diaries of the participants and not allowed to be cancelled for more 'important' matters.

The next stage is to *plan* the content. This might mean the social worker giving her supervisor a case file to read prior to their meeting or for the latter to draw up an agenda of issues that they wish to raise. There seems little point in trying to decide what you want to talk about when you actually get together and suggests neither party will be taking seriously the session. Forethought and planning lead to best use of available time in any aspect of social work and midwifery too I'm sure, so the same principle should be applied to supervision. Honest and open communication leads to the truth being told so full *participation* is the next component.

We learn best from situations when we have the opportunity to *peruse* them and so in supervision the worker and manager should consider what was said and reflect retrospectively as well as at the time, on what occurred.

The pay off should be the social worker being able to *perform* in an improved, effective and efficient manner.

PURPOSE - PROGRAMME - PLAN - PARTICIPATE - PERUSE- PERFORM

It is the manager's responsibility to initiate the discussion of the purpose with a new member of staff and establish ground rules about confidentiality - accountability - action, so that agreement is reached about the purpose of supervision. Programming, Planning and Participation are shared responsibilities with the Perusal and Performance aspects resting with the social worker assisted by the manager's support.

The Frank Sinatra section – 'I did it my way'

My 17 years experience as recipient and provider of supervision in a variety of conditions leads me to the following suggestion as a model of supervision.

Having taken on board the previous six points – the '6 Ps' – supervision of a social worker with an active case load should be held *fortnightly with alternate sessions focusing on the Managerial and Professional issues.*

The managerial session would use a caseload measurement system as discussed earlier. Even then when I have used one in supervision I always commenced the session with a question to the social worker about how they felt in relation to their workload. Did they feel under pressure or were they coping all right with the amount of work?

Would they say they were busy or, heaven forbid, slack and able to take another case – this being a very rare scenario! A managerial session would then look at each case allocated to the social worker. Frequency of visiting was recorded, this being a crucial component of the measurement system. Other factors which were part of the measurement systemwere noted e.g. sessions as Duty Officer, training commitments, regular time tabled meetings.

Work undertaken would be reviewed and plans made for future contact. If there were statutory reviews coming up then reports would be written and read prior to the event. There would be follow up to any case conferences and I would make sure the decisions were being implemented.

All decisions would be recorded with a summary of the discussion. The social worker received a copy for the client file and the manager kept a copy for the file containing a record of supervision with the member of staff.

Cases would be closed, if closing summaries had been written and a caseload measurement figure finalized and agreed.

Managerial supervision would end with a reflection on whether the case load measurement and discussion had validated the workers feelings about how busy they were. Usually this was the case.

The professional session would be based on one or more cases that the social worker or I wished to focus on. This might be prior to a case conference or a court hearing. It could be to reflect on a piece of good practice or learn from a traumatic or challenging one.

Implicit is the shared understanding that both participants are engaged in a learning process. This is not one sided as the manager will be utilizing and improving (hopefully) management and supervisory skills at the same time as the social worker benefits from the process of being supervised.

The professional session gives the opportunity to raise issues about the worker's developmental needs and career progression. Training needs would be identified and agreement reached on how these can be pursued.

Scope would be given for the social worker to raise any work related issue pertinent to themselves. Time at the end should be allowed for any other competent business.

Informal or on-shift management

Within social work a manager will be providing supervision for staff during the day as they go about their lawful business. This goes on between social workers and their managers all the time usually prefaced with the question, 'have you got a moment?' or 'could I have a quick word?'

Be assured that as a manager it is worthwhile making that moment available.

As a manager and supervisor I have to be available for staff to consult with me, respond to their queries and be decisive in my actions. I have to make sure that all procedures are adhered to and proper professional standards are maintained.

In essence the role is one of leadership and exercising responsibility for the actions of staff on duty. I am manager and professional supervisor at the same time. The split between managerial and professional blurs in the demands made on me and on the staff. Time for reflection in formal supervision off shift is essential and allows us to sort out any disagreements, misunderstandings or just plain mistakes made whilst on shift.

In the Emergency Duty Team we do not do a lot of trivial stuff as the work is all emergencies and crisis intervention. The need for open and honest communication is paramount and I'm back where I started about the prerequisites for good supervision.

Conclusion

It may be that something in this paper has rung a bell with you. Either 'that's a good idea' or 'that sounds like the writer is deranged'. My feeling is that some of the things I have said will be applicable to you as midwives. Could you benefit from regular, planned supervision with a clear and open agenda? Would it help to have a caseload measurement system which records how much you do and how busy you are? Is supervision something that can encapsulate management and professional considerations and if so how is that best facilitated? Is it possible to meet with your supervisor and discuss management issues in a separate session to one focused on your professional performance and developmental needs.

I feel confident that I have highlighted the basics of good supervision. I will not repeat the '6 Ps' but I will finish by highlighting the positive and negative outcomes of supervision.

On the negative side of the equation, if you are afraid of being truthful and open in supervision what can one hope to achieve?

When supervision is an event that is perceived as being critical and a fault finding exercise, who will benefit? If you only see your supervisor when something goes wrong, what is the basis for your relationship?

Positive supervision will be regular and have an agenda founded on open and honest communication. It will be professional and supportive within an acknowledged management structure as both parties participate in the functional side of the process.

For supervision is a process not a personal matter. The relationship between manager and worker should be safe yet challenging in order to facilitate good practice.

It is no use us pretending or bemoaning the fact that your boss has to be – how can I put it in a politically correct phrase – a Jekyll and Hyde? (or has to be to you both Virginia Bottomley and Caroline Flint!)

A manager has to be supportive to staff but must be able to manage their performance in a way that ensures professional and satisfactory standards are maintained.

Managers should, by their experience and skills, be able to assess performance, give guidance and then be accountable and responsible for the actions of those whom they supervise. You cannot achieve this by jumping up and down when something goes wrong or blaming staff for their mistakes if you have not been monitoring their performance and giving feedback in regular supervision.

Supervision can go wrong and be a disaster for all concerned. I have anecdotal evidence from my career which would make you cringe. Importantly the majority of my experience of supervision either as recipient or provider has been positive and beneficial.

Probably I should rephrase the last sentence to delete recipient and provider replacing them with *participant*. Good supervision is not something you have done to you or do to others but involves both parties participating in the process of a working relationship.

Supervision of Midwives in 1995

Glynnis Mayes
Assistant Director, Midwifery Supervision and Practice English National Board for Nursing, Midwifery and Health Visiting

Introduction

Supervision of midwives has developed more during the last five years than at any other time since its inception. These changes have been initiated at all levels of the process from the United Kingdom Central Council (UKCC), the National Boards, the Local Supervising Authorities (LSAs) to the supervisors of midwives establishing local systems. This paper will outline some of the features of supervision of midwives as it is being put into practice in England at the present time.

Supervision of midwives by midwives for midwives

It is fitting for the midwifery profession to scrutinize and develop recommendations for the way forward in supervision at this time of change, when more is being demanded of midwives in their practice, and expectations of the supervisors' role are rising. Since the prime objective of supervision is to enable midwives to practise competently and confidently within the statutory framework, it is important that the future of supervision of midwives should be determined, shaped and led by midwives.

Recent developments in the arrangements for supervision have been instigated by the following bodies:

The UKCC

The UKCC Midwifery Committee has had a major influence through the way that the statutory framework and standards have been developed (Roch, 1995).

The Midwives Rules (1993) incorporate amendments arising from the Nurses, Midwives and Health Visitors Act, 1992. Rule 45 specifies new standards for LSAs, requiring them to publish details of how the process of supervision operates within the Region. This enables greater consistency, clarifies for midwives what to expect from the process and for supervisors what is expected of them.

The Midwife's Code of Practice (1994) sets out the standards required for midwifery practice and for the effective contribution of supervision. The supervisor of midwives is required to provide each midwife with 'support as a colleague, counsellor and adviser' and to 'promote positive working relationships' in order to fulfil the 'common aim of optimum care for mothers and babies'. Each supervisor should supervise no more than 40 practising midwives and must have completed appropriate preparation for the role. It is also recommended that the LSA function should be discharged by a practising midwife.

A task group has been set up to review the statutory supervision of midwives and submit recommendations for consideration by Council for future guidance on standards. This work has been informed by the results of a survey of all supervisors and LSAs in the UK, and the outcomes of a conference held in October 1994 of representatives of the statutory bodies, LSAs and lead supervisors.

The English National Board

Through its statutory remit to provide advice and guidance to LSAs, the Board regards supervision of midwives as crucial to developing midwifery practice. The Board's strategy for strengthening supervision has involved a programme of initiatives, building on the foundations of the work begun by the late Anne Stewart (Page and Thomas, 1995).

The programmes of preparation for supervisors of midwives developed by the Board and provided by the LSAs in conjunction with colleges of midwifery education, ensure that supervisors develop expertise to equip them for their complex role. The courses focus on a pro-active approach to supporting midwifery practice and are structured around the Board's open learning pack, (ENB, 1992) which provides a common basis for supervision of midwives throughout the country.

Continuing education for supervisors has been reviewed by the Board and the statutory follow-up courses are planned as a progression from the initial programme of preparation, building upon those learning outcomes and expertise.

The Board has regular contact with LSAs through meetings with LSA representatives at the Board, visits to the LSAs and in providing advice on specific issues. This has enabled a more consistent approach to be achieved throughout the country in developing systems for supervision. Currently, the Board is working with the LSAs on their proposals for the transfer of the LSA function in order to ensure that robust frameworks for effective supervision are established.

Local Supervising Authorities

Considerable work has been undertaken by LSAs in updating and revising the policies and protocols in the light of current developments. Standards for supervision have been drawn up by all LSAs and local arrangements are being audited in relation to these standards in order to identify examples of good practice as well as problem areas. As a result of this, together with suggestions from midwives locally, many units are developing innovative systems for supervision appropriate for the midwives' practice needs.

The Royal College of Midwives

The Royal College of Midwives (RCM) has formed a council working group on supervision as a direct result of a resolution passed at its 1994 Annual General Meeting. The focus of the work includes the role of the LSA and selection criteria for the nomination and appointment of supervisors of midwives. The group aims to produce a RCM position statement for the profession specifying minimum criteria and standards.

The Association of Radical Midwives

The ARM has had concerns for some years about the controlling and negative effects of supervision on midwives' practice. This has been pursued in the journal 'Midwifery Matters' (ARM, 1994) and the national conference at which the papers in this volume were presented.

Current features and developments in supervision of midwives in England

The approach to supervision

Perhaps the most fundamental (and necessary!) development has been the change in approach which many supervisors of midwives are now adopting (ENB, 1995). Examples of oppressive or ineffectual supervision are still vivid memories for those midwives who were on the receiving end and those experiences provide the evidence of the inadequacy of such approaches in stimulating professional growth and innovative practice. Developments in the framework for supervision, the LSA protocols, national standards and the thorough preparation for the role have enabled supervisors of midwives to form a much clearer understanding of their role, its purpose and objectives.

Originally, supervision of midwives was set up as a vital component of the professional regulation of midwives in protecting the public. Through the 1902 Midwives Act, the Central Midwives Board was established to draw up the regulations for safe practice and the LSAs carried the responsibility for ensuring that these regulations were met at a time when the majority of midwives practised independently. Today, through the Nurses, Midwives and Health Visitors Act, it is the UKCC which formulates the Rules and standards of professional practice to safeguard the interests of the public. The LSAs are still responsible for establishing the framework to enable the statutory requirements to be fulfilled and to take appropriate action if the Rules are breached.

The focus of the supervisor of midwives, however, is moving away from inspection and seeking out non-compliance with the Rules with the subsequent reporting to the LSA.

The supervisor's overriding purpose is to enable midwives to practise competently by supporting them to take responsibility for their professional practice (Mayes, 1995). The aim is to prevent poor practice and therefore to avoid midwives being reported to the statutory body unless there is no means of rectifying the difficulty to ensure safe practice in the future.

Supervision of midwives is assuming a more prominent profile particularly as the numbers of midwifery management posts are dwindling. Increasingly, supervisors are exploring ways of strengthening professional leadership for midwives, by creating an environment where midwives can undertake their full role and responsibilities, where professional practice is supported by appropriate protocols and policies and there are appropriate support services and mechanisms. Access to the supervisor by individual midwives is being promoted to encourage midwives to talk through issues and dilemmas of their practice, to determine how to resolve any problems and to learn from their experience.

In some units, supervisors hold regular meetings with midwives to discuss topical practice issues and to clarify how midwives can benefit from the supervisory process. Some supervisors hold regular 'surgeries' for midwives to meet them. Many have set up a central resource file and notice board with essential information, while others have provided information folders for all midwives. The planned annual meeting between each midwife and her supervisor is now well established in the majority of services and is proving to be of benefit both to the midwife and the service. As a two-way process, discussion focuses on the midwife's professional needs and also her achievements and ideas for new developments.

With the implementation of initiatives associated with woman-centred care (Expert Maternity Group, 1993) midwives are gradually taking on the responsibilities of the lead professional, of providing midwife-led care and supporting women in exercising choice. With these changes in practice, the midwife's accountability becomes a prominent issue. Continuity of care and carer brings continuity of responsibility, very different from the 'institutionalized' involvement of ward-based midwives. In exercising choice, the woman may opt for a style of care which is inconsistent with Trust policy or which may be unfamiliar to the midwife or may even carry potential risks. How is the midwife to respond, when she is accountable for 'safeguarding the interests and well-being of patients and clients', for 'acknowledging any limitations in knowledge and competence and declining any duties or responsibilities unless able to perform them in a safe and skilled manner'? (Code of Professional Conduct, UKCC 1992)

When facing such dilemmas, the midwife has access to the supervisor of midwives to discuss a plan of action or the outcome of the discussions with the mother. The supervisor is in the best position to negotiate for the Trust to authorize exceptional arrangements for care when specifically requested by the mother. She may also be able to mobilize appropriate support for a midwife undertaking a home confinement in difficult circumstances (Mayes, 1995).

Selection and appointment of supervisors of midwives
The role of the supervisor of midwives is a complex one and to be effective the supervisor must be both credible in her professional judgement, approachable and acceptable to the midwives in order to gain their trust and to be used as a resource to support their practice. The credibility is dependent on possessing a wide knowledge base together with relevant experience of current midwifery practice in order to make decisions based on recognized evidence and to contribute to wider issues concerning maternity services. The ability to relate well to the midwives requires good inter-

personal skills and an intimate understanding of the situations and conditions which midwives face in their day-to-day practice. It is essential therefore, that the right people are appointed as supervisors of midwives.

Rule 44 of the UKCC Midwives Rules specifies the qualifications for supervisors. The skills and knowledge are acquired and demonstrated by assessment on the course of preparation. The acceptability to the local midwives is an aspect which can be addressed through the system for nomination and selection. Since the appointment of supervisors is made by the LSA and not the employer, the process has differed from the usual recruitment and selection systems for NHS posts. Until quite recently it had been customary for the existing supervisor to nominate a suitable candidate when a vacancy arose and the nomination confirmed by the LSA. This is now changing quite significantly.

Increasingly, vacancies for supervisors of midwives are being notified to all local midwives, together with information about the role and essential criteria for selection. Midwives interested in being considered are invited for an informal discussion and to submit an application for competitive interview. In some units, midwives are invited to nominate midwives whom they consider would be suitable and these are then short-listed for interview. The final appointment is then subject to successful completion of the course of preparation.

There are approximately 800 supervisors of midwives practising in England. Currently, there is a significant turnover arising, in part, from the management restructuring within Trusts and provider units. In many districts it has been decided to increase the number of supervisors to achieve a more favourable ratio of supervisors to midwives. As a result, the demand for places on the courses of preparation has exceeded the initial predictions, and to date, supervisors who have completed the new programmes of preparation comprise 30 per cent of total complement in England. They, therefore, form a significant proportion and locally they contribute their new perspective to the experience of the existing supervisors. The local teams are also enriched by the range of expertise and backgrounds of the members. Of those supervisors who have completed the new courses, the areas of practice are represented as follows:

Clinical practice	44 per cent
Midwifery Management	37 per cent
Other (research and practice development)	9 per cent
Not known	7 per cent
Midwifery education	3 per cent

(ENB, 1995).

The midwife and her supervisor

In the vast majority of services, each midwife is linked to a named supervisor but also has open access to any of the other supervisors of midwives locally (ENB, 1995). There are a variety of models for allocation of supervisors, ranging from the supervisor who also carries managerial responsibility, random allocation, each supervisor having a mixed caseload of hospital and community midwives, to a growing trend for mid-wives to choose their supervisor. Midwives practising independently, and many mid-wife teachers, notify their intention to practise to a number of supervisors, but identify one with whom they have the closest contact, to discuss their practice and plan their professional development activities. In many units, when the allocation of the named supervisor has been confirmed, an introductory meeting takes place between the midwife and her supervisor to establish the 'ground rules' and expectations of the relationship and how the process will operate (ENB, 1995).

The one aspect where the supportive colleague and counsellor relationship, as pro-moted in the UKCCs Midwife's Code of Practice, may break down is the rare event of an incident involving poor practice. Even if the case is not reported to the LSA, it is not easy for any midwife to accept criticism of her practice, particularly if her actions are blamed as the cause of poor outcomes for the mother and baby. With the emotional stress, she is unlikely to be at her most receptive to formal advice from her supervisor of midwives however necessary this may be. It is made even worse if the midwife does not agree with the judgement of the supervisor. For this reason, it is essential for the supervisor's credibility that she is able to base her decisions on sound evidence researched in current practice and that she listens carefully to the midwife's view.

The approach which the supervisor takes is therefore critical in influencing the extent to which the midwife is able to learn from the incident and improve her practice in the future. The supervisor has to be highly skilled to achieve a positive outcome in which the midwife still feels valued and respected for the good aspects of her practice and is motivated to work on the weaker areas. Throughout the process, the midwife must be assured that she has access to other supervisors of midwives, either within or outside the unit, who are not involved with the investigation.

Conclusion

As a dynamic process, supervision of midwives is changing as the practice of mid-wives and their professional needs are changing. These changes are taking place at an ever increasing pace, as identified in the practice visits to maternity services under-taken by the Board's Midwifery Specialist Officers.

Supervision of midwives has a history of being poorly understood and evident only when an untoward incident occurs. Sadly, it is mainly the examples of poor supervi-sion which are remembered and the skilled, effective actions by supervisors, with a wealth of experience, have been taken for granted or gone unnoticed. Considerable work has been invested in developing supervision over the last decade and this has been directed towards both addressing the inadequacies of the past and also exploit-ing its potential for the future. Supervisors of midwives are becoming involved in advising for purchasing and the process of supervision is being viewed as a valuable component of quality assurance, clinical audit and risk management. The expertise of supervisors emerging from the new courses of preparation is most evident in their enthusiasm for empowering and providing support for midwives to enable them to practise as confident, competent professionals who instil confidence in the women in their care.

References

Association of Radical Midwives (1994). 'First draft proposals for future midwifery supervision'. *Midwifery Matters*, Issue 60 pp.26–27.

Department of Health (1993). *Changing Childbirth: Report of the Expert Maternity Group*. London: HMSO.

English National Board for Nursing, Midwifery and Health Visiting (1992). *Preparation of Supervisors of Midwives*. London: ENB.

English National Board for Nursing, Midwifery and Health Visiting (1995). *Development in Midwifery Education and Practice*. London: ENB.

Mayes, G. (1995). *Supervisors of Midwives - How can we facilitate change, in The Challenge of Changing Childbirth Midwifery Educational Resource Pack*. London: ENB.

Page, L., Thomas, M. (1995). 'The English National Board' *British Journal of Midwifery* 3 (4) April 1995, pp.217–219.

Roch, S (1995). 'Statutory regulations: What's in it for midwives?' *British Journal of Midwifery* 3 (4) April 1995, pp.203–205.

United Kingdom Central Council for Nursing, Midwifery and Health Visiting (1994**)**. *The Midwives Code of Practice*. London: UKCC.

United Kingdom Central Council for Nursing, Midwifery and Health Visiting (1993). *Midwives' Rules*. London: UKCC.

United Kingdom Central Council for Nursing, Midwifery and Health Visiting (1992). *Code of Professional Conduct*. London: UKCC.

Recommendations of Discussion Groups

1. *Selection*

What factors should be taken into consideration when considering the selection (and de-selection) of midwifery supervisors? How and by whom should potential supervisors be nominated? Should there be a fixed term of office followed by re-selection or de-selection? Should midwives have some part in selection of supervisors? Should supervisors supervise working colleagues or supervise midwives in other areas?

Conclusion: Supervisors should be selected for their personal characteristics. There should be nominations of supervisors from different disciplines than the Supervisor. Supervisors should understand the role. Midwives should be asked for their support. Every five years there should be re-selection. Supervisors should not supervise more than 20 Midwives and could be from another practice area. Supervisors could be of a higher grade but there was some discussion over the election of Midwives and maintaining the standard of care.

2. *Preparation and education*

Appraise current preparation (e.g. ENB Distance Learning Course) and suggest improvements and alternatives if necessary. Draw up five points.

Conclusion: Early preparation of personal and professional development in their basic education as midwives. Selected Supervisors need to be able to demonstrate this – e.g. interpersonal skills, negotiating skills, teaching skills, political awareness, education needs to be moving forward. Need to strongly demonstrate that they are our advocate for women and Midwives, being open, flexible and approachable. We see the ENB Distance Learning Course as a transmitter. Reports are that the pack has been really beneficial in contrast to the three day course. Suggestions were made that more interaction with the pack is important to increase learning. The pack needs continuous development with more use of refreshers, up-dating current supervisors and Audit Supervisors need to support and be supported. (N.B. stress and long hours). The future of the role was debated. Midwifery is changing in the field of ownership and practice.

3. *Communication*

Consider the channels of communication, between supervisors and midwives, between supervisors and management and between supervisors and other supervisors. How can this be improved?

Conclusion: *Supervisor: Midwife*
1. Open door policy
2. Wide understanding of what a supervisor is there for
3. Named supervisor with the right to change, right of access to another
4. In a supervisory investigation, the two elements of supervision should be fulfilled by separate individuals
5. Audit – evaluation of supervisors activities
6. 24 hour supervisory advice and access. All midwives should know how to contact them.

Supervisors: General Management
1. Regular meetings
2. Management understanding of the role of the supervisors
3. Contracts recognize the authority, value and purpose of supervision
4. Supervising input into policy and risk management
5. Supervisors consulted on ALL midwifery issues.

Supervisor: Supervisor
1. Regular meetings – local and regional LSA. One to one basis as necessary
2. Access to link supervisors
3. All supervisors have a right to attend all LSA supervisory meetings
4. Publish anonymized supervisory investigation results.

Very important: Channels of communication between supervisors of Midwifery and Approved Midwifery Teachers and other educationalists.

4. *Conflicting roles of 'policeman' and 'friend'*
The midwifery supervisor has two responsibilities:

1. To protect the public against bad practitioners
2. To guide and befriend midwives under supervision.

Can these two potentially conflicting roles be reconciled in one person? If so, suggest ways in which both roles can be safeguarded against each other. If not, suggest alternatives.

Conclusion: The term policing was rejected. There was some feeling of negativity. There should be a change in clinical supervision with the public image needing to be raised. Midwives need to have had it made clear on what basis they are approaching the supervisor – policeman or friend. Ideally, the role of the supervisor is one of guide and friend. When investigations or disciplinary issues are raised, another supervisor should take on this role.

5. *Clinical credibility*

If a supervisor of midwives has a clinical caseload, does this enhance the role? If so, how should the caseload be assessed? How can teachers, researches and other non-clinical midwives be supervisors?

Conclusion: Clinical caseloads do not necessarily enhance supervisory roles. We need supervisors with a mixture of experience and expertise. Midwives should be able to question credibility. Supervisors from other areas may be appropriate but with supervision of new Midwives from within their own ranks.

6. *Accountability*

To whom should the supervisor be accountable? How can impartiality be ensured? Should supervision be a job in its own right rather than an extra role tagged on to a management post? How are supervision duties assessed and paid for? Who pays for supervision? What input should service users have? Who sets the ratio of supervisors to midwives? What changes should be made to all these aspects of supervision?

Conclusion: Ideally ...

1. The supervisor should be visibly accountable to both the LSA at Health Commission/Consortium level and to the midwife for practice in accordance with agreed national standards which are audited annually.

2. The Health Commission/Consortium funds the LSA post which should be a Midwife. Purchasers will require that providers pay the midwives for their supervisory role as specified in contracts which are advised on by the MSLC. (Ratio of Midwives to Supervisor = 1:30)

3. The midwife should be able to choose a named supervisor who is not her line manger.

This concluded the Conference proceedings, with discussion limited to between delegates only, as comments from the floor.

The Chair thanked the various speakers, helpers and organizers and officially closed the Conference.

Bibliography

Allison, J. (1995). *Personal Communication.*

Association of Radical Midwives (1993). 'Report of the spring national meeting' *Midwifery Matters,* No. 57 Summer pp.27-28.

Association of Radical Midwives (1994). 'Future midwifery supervision' *Midwifery Matters,* No. 60 Spring pp.25-27.

Association of Supervisors of Midwives (1992). *Supervision – The Whys and Wherefores.* Great Yarmouth: ASM.

Beech, B.A.L. (1993). 'We told you so, birth at home and the Mental Health Act' *AIMS Journal,* Vol. 6, No. 3, pp.10-12.

Beech, B.A.L. (1993). 'Guidelines for home birth' *AIMS Journal,* Vol. 5 No. 2, pp. 4-7.

Beech, B.A.L. (1993). 'Supervision of midwives'. *AIMS Journal,* Vol 5:2 pp.1-3.

Bent, A. (1995). *Personal Communication.*

Brammer, L.M., Wasserman, A.C. (1977). 'Supervision in counselling and psychotherapy'. In Kurpius, D.J. *Training.* Wewstport, Connecticut: Greenwood Press.

British Association for Counselling Resources Directory 1991. British Association for Counselling, 1 Regent Place, Rugby CV21 2PJ.

Butterworth, C.A., Faugier J. (1992). *Clinical Supervision and Mentorship in Nursing,* London: Chapman and Hall.

Crainer, S. (1988). 'Making boss-power positive.' *The Sunday Times* 9th October

Cumberledge Report (1993). *Changing Childbirth The Report of the Expert Maternity Group.* London: HMSO.

Daft, R.L. (1992). *Organization Theory and Design.* 2nd Ed. New York: West Publishing Co.

Davis, K. (1994). 'Is statutory supervision central to our professional identity?' *British Journal of Midwifery,* Vol. 2, No. 7, pp.304-05.

Department of Health (1993). *Changing Childbirth: Report of the Expert Maternity Group.* London: HMSO.

Department of Health (1994). *Clinical Audit in the Nursing and Therapy Professions.* London: HMSO.

Department of Health (1994). *The Challenges for Nursing and Midwifery in the 21st century.* London: HMSO.

Department of Trade and Industry (1991). *Total Quality Management and Effective Leadership.* London: HMSO.

Donnison, J. (1977). *Midwives and Medical Men.* London: Heinemann.

Duff, E. (1994). 'Meeting Report: UKCC Working Conference on Supervision of Midwifery' *Midwives Chronicle and Nursing Notes,* Vol.107. No.1282. November pp. 434-435.

English National Board (1992). *Preparation of Supervisors of Midwives: An Open Learning Programme.* London: ENB.

English National Board (1995). *Development in Midwifery Education and Practice.* London: ENB.

Ferguson, P. (1994). 'RCM Annual Conference 1994 Report' *Midwives Chronicle and Nursing Notes,* Vol. 107, No. 1280 p.341.

Flint, C. (1988). 'On the brink, midwifery in britain' In Kitzinger, S. (Ed.) *The Midwife Challenge.* p.32.

Flint, C. (1988). 'The Golden Thread', *Association of Radical Midwives Magazine* No. 37, p.18-19.

Ford, K., Jones, A. (1987). *Student Supervision.* Basingstoke: MacMillan.

Hawkins, P., Shohet, R. (1989). *Supervision in the Helping Professions.* Buckingham: Open University Press.

Heagerty, B.V. (1990). *Gender and Professionalization: The Struggle for British Midwifery 1900–1936.* Unpublished Phd thesis, Michigan State University. (copy in RCM library, London)

HMSO (1982). *Report from the Select Committee on the Registration of Midwives, House of Commons.* London: HMSO.

House of Commons (1979). *Nurses, Midwives and Health Visitors Act.* London: HMSO.

Huczynski, A., Buchanan, D. (1991). *Organizational Behaviour - An Introductory Test.* (2nd Ed). New York: Prentice Hall.

Isherwood, K (1988). 'Friend or watchdog?' *Nursing Times* 84:24 June 15th. p.65.

Jenkins, R. (1995). *The Law and Midwifery.* Oxford: Blackwell.

Keane, H. (1995). 'The waterbirth experience, a supervisor's perspective' *Midwives,* January, pp.9-11.

Landsell, M. (1989). 'Friend and Counsellor', *Nursing Times* 85 (28), p.86.

Leap, N., Hunter, B. (1993). *The Midwife's Tale.* London: Scarlet Press.

Logue, M. (1990). 'Management of the third stage of labour. A midwife's view' *Journal of Obstetrics and Gynaecology* 10, Suppl. 2, S10-S12.

Mayes, G. (1995). 'Supervisors of midwives - how can we facilitate change', in *The Challenge of Changing Childbirth Midwifery Educational Resource Pack.* London: ENB.

McFeeley, M.D. (1988). *Lady Inspectors.* Oxford: Blackwell.

Mintzberg, H (1991). 'The effective organization, forces and forms', *Sloan Management Review* Winter pp.54-67.

Nursing Notes archives kept in RCM library London.

Page, L. (1995). 'Effective group practice in midwifery' In: Page, L. (Ed.) *Working with Women,* Oxford: Blackwell Science.

Page, L., Thomas, M. (1995). 'The English National Board' *British Journal of Midwifery* 3 (4) April, pp.217-219.

Platt-Koch, L.M. (1986). 'Clinical Supervision for psychiatric nurses'. *Journal of Psychological Nursing.* 26; 1; pp.7-15.

Robinson, J. (1995). 'Emily's choice' *AIMS Journal,* Vol. 7 No. 1, pp. 4-5.

Roch, S (1995). 'Statutory regulations: What's in it for midwives?' *British Journal of Midwifery* 3 (4) April, pp.203-205.

Royal College of Midwives (1991). *Report of the Royal College of Midwives Commission on Legislation Relating to Midwives.* London: RCM.

Smith, F.B (1979). *The People's Health.* London: Croom Helm.

Smith, J. (1994). 'We told you so'. *AIMS Journal* 6:3 pp.10-12.

Stewart, R. (1963). *The Reality of Management*. London: Pan Books.

Taylor, M. (1994). The Supervision of Midwives' *Midwifery Matters* No. 60 Spring p.28.

Thomas, P. (1994). 'Accountable for what?' *AIMS Journal,* Vol. 6 No. 3, pp.1–5.

UKCC (1990). *The Report of the Post Registration Education and Practice Project*. London: UKCC.

UKCC (1992a). *Code of Professional Conduct*. London: UKCC.

UKCC (1993). *The Council's Position Concerning a Period of Support and Preceptorship*. (Registrar's Letter 1/1993.) London: UKCC.

UKCC (1993). *Midwives Rules*. London: UKCC.

UKCC (1994). *A Midwife's Code of Practice*. London: UKCC.

UKCC (1992). *Code of Professional Conduct*. London: UKCC.

Walton, I., Hamilton, M. (1995). *Midwives and Changing Childbirth*. Hale: Books for Midwives Press.

Wilde, C. (1984). 'See Me In My Office' *Association of Radical Midwives* No.23.

Witz, A. (1992). *Professions and Patriarchy*. London: Routledge.

Who are the Association of Radical Midwives?

The Association of Radical Midwives are midwives and student midwives who believe in the National Health Service and are committed to improving the maternity care provided by the NHS. They strongly believe that all women have the right to a service tailored more closely to their needs and to a sympathetic attitude on the part of their professional attendants.

ARM is primarily a support group for those having difficulty in getting or giving good, sympathetic, personalized midwifery care. Associate membership of ARM is offered to non-midwives and groups concerned with the improvements in the maternity service. A few ARM members are working independently outside the NHS.

What changes do ARM seek?

ARM seek to re-establish the confidence of the midwife in her own skills, to share ideas, skills and information and to encourage midwives in their support of women's active participation in birth. They also seek to reaffirm the need for midwives to provide continuity of care, to explore alternative patterns of care and to encourage the evaluation of developments within the sphere of midwifery practice.

How did ARM start?

In 1976 two student midwives from different hospitals met and shared their frustration and disappointment with the increasing trend towards medicalization and intervention as opposed to the true midwifery they had come to the UK to learn. They met regularly for mutual support and study, others joined them, and following publication in a national newspaper of an article about the group, they were overwhelmed by the sympathetic response from midwives all over the country. Today ARM has regional groups in every part of the UK, as well as a number of overseas members. Many midwifery schools and medical libraries subscribe regularly, making *Midwifery Matters* a familiar journal on the shelves.

What has ARM done so far?

ARM has been pro-active on many issues which threaten midwifery and good maternity care, campaigning and lobbying in support of an enhanced service within the NHS for childbearing women, as well as a stronger professional identity for midwives. ARM is consulted by Government departments and other bodies on midwifery issues and the Association was invited to submit evidence to the Government Health Committee during the 1991/92 enquiry into maternity services in the UK.

In 1986, after two years of intensive research, ARM published their proposals for the future of the maternity services, which were called *The Vision*. This report has been used as a basis for many innovatory changes in maternity care throughout the UK. The philosophy of the document, and of the Association, is that every pregnant woman should be cared for by a small number of professionals, giving her the opportunity to get to know and trust her attendants and raising the standard of her care by the continuity thus provided. One of the Working Parties split off from ARM and became an independent registered charity in order to obtain funding for a Midwives Information and Resources Service. It is well known today as MIDIRS, which produces regular digests of worldwide midwifery based information and has also set up the world's first midwifery database for the use of researchers in midwifery related topics.

The ARM leaflet 'What is a midwife' explains the role of a midwife and explodes popular myths. Thanks to sponsorship ARM are able to offer free supplies for distribution in antenatal clinics, women's groups, health centres, etc.

What next for ARM?

Research into midwifery-related issues is growing and using these studies ARM are encouraging the awareness of choices in maternity care, at present only available to the more assertive woman. ARM works towards a future in which these choices will be freely offered to every woman by the health professionals involved in her care. ARM welcomes all who wish to join them in this work – come and enjoy the support and friendship of like-minded people with a common aim.

ARM support their work largely by subscriptions from members. For an annual fee members receive the quarterly journal *Midwifery Matters*, pay reduced entrance fees at ARM national meetings and study days and may borrow books and videos from ARM library free of charge. Subscriptions may begin at any time and cost £22 (UK), £30 (overseas) and £11 (Optional concession, unwaged, grant-aided students, etc) p.a.

For further information please contact:
Ishbel Karger
ASSOCIATION OF RADICAL MIDWIVES
62 Greetby Hill
Ormskirk
Lancashire L39 2DT
Tel: 01695 572776

Books for Midwives Press

Books for Midwives Press, in joint collaboration with the Royal College of Midwives, publish books written by experts in the midwifery field to meet the practical needs of the working midwife and midwifery student. Below is a list of our current and forthcoming titles:

Current titles

A Short History of Clinical Midwifery	Philip Rhodes	£17.95
Communicating Midwifery	Caroline Flint	£12.95
Teaching Physical Skill for the Childbearing Year	Eileen Brayshaw & Pauline Wright	£10.95
HIV Infection in Pregnancy	Caroline Shepherd	£ 6.95
Antenatal Investigations	Maureen Boyle	£ 6.95
Understanding Obstetric Ultrasound	Jean Proud	£10.95
MIRIAD	NPEU	£14.95
Aquanatal Exercises	Gillian Hawksworth	£ 6.95
Holding On?	Hazel McHaffie	£ 9.95
Reactions to Motherhood	Jean Ball	£10.95
Sexuality and Motherhood	Irene Walton	£10.95
Legal Aspects of Midwifery	Bridgit Dimond	£12.95
Midwives and 'Changing Childbirth'	Walton & Hamilton	£ 9.95
Waterbirth	Dianne Garland	£10.95
The Pregnant Drug Addict	Catherine Siney	£ 9.95

If you would like to receive details about future titles and be placed on our mailing list, please send your details to the address given below.

Please order *Books for Midwives Press* titles from your usual bookseller and encourage them to stock midwifery titles. If you prefer you can order from us by sending a cheque (made payable to *Books for Midwives Press*) to the address below or by telephoning 0161-929-0929 for credit/debit card orders (Access/Visa/Switch/Delta). For overseas postage please add 25% of total price. All UK orders are sent postage free.

Please send orders or requests for catalogues/information to:

BOOKS FOR MIDWIVES PRESS
Freepost WA1836
Hale
Cheshire
WA15 9BR
0161 929 0929